The Dental Amputee

The Dental Amputee

Professor David Harris

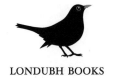

LONDUBH BOOKS

First published in 2015

by Londubh Books

18 Casimir Avenue, Harold's Cross, Dublin 6w, Ireland

www.londubh.ie

1 3 5 4 2

Origination by Londubh Books; cover by sinédesign

Printed by ScandBook AB, Falun, Sweden

ISBN: 978-1-907535-10-9

A Note on the Text

This book is set in Adobe Garamond Pro, Gotham Rounded and Helvetica.

Professor Per-Ingvar Brånemark
3 May 1929-20 December 2014

This book is dedicated to the life and memory of the father of modern dental implants, Professor Per-Ingvar Brånemark, a most remarkable scientist, clinician, innovater, philosopher, mentor and friend.

About the Author

Professor David Harris was born in Ireland and is a specialist oral surgeon. Having qualified in dentistry in the Royal College of Surgeons in Ireland, he subsequently completed medical studies in University College Hospital, London. He became a Fellow of the Faculty of Dental Surgery in the Royal College of Surgeons of England and was awarded a Fellowship of the Faculty of Dentistry in the Royal College of Surgeons in Ireland.

In 1983 he introduced osseointegrated implants into his clinical practice to help patients who had lost all their teeth. As a member of one of a small number of international pioneer teams working with Per-Ingvar Brånemark from Sweden, 'the father of modern dental implants', he was the first clinician to utilise these implants in private practice in the UK or Ireland. He holds academic and teaching appointments as an associate professor in Trinity College Dublin and as a visiting professor to the Medical University of Warsaw. He maintains a private practice in the Blackrock Clinic, Dublin, where he is a consultant and Clinical Director of Blackrock Clinic Specialist Dentistry.

David has lectured extensively and provides postgraduate courses internationally. A founder member of the European Association for Osseointegration, he has served as president of the association on two occasions. He has contributed chapters on the topic of dental implants in three international textbooks as well as contributing original research and articles to several scientific journals.

For further information please see: www.blackrockclinicdental.ie or email david@drdavidharris.com.

Acknowledgements

In writing this book I have relied on and benefitted from the help, advice and encouragement received from many people.

First of all I must thank Terry Prone for encouraging me to write a book on this topic for the general public and for her constant help and advice.

Thanks also:

To my publisher in Londubh Books, Jo O'Donoghue, for her infinite patience, understanding and guidance; to my colleagues in Blackrock Clinic Specialist Dentistry, Dr Michael Freedman, Dr Una Lally and Dr Lewis Winning, for their ongoing support and critical contributions; a warm thanks to Barbro Brånemark for her review, encouragement and help; to Dr Seamus Sharkey and Dr Wolfgang Bolz for their most helpful and thoughtful reviews; to Paul Harris for all his help and expertise with the illustrations and assistance in obtaining copyright permissions; and to Lia Cowan for her artistic skills in providing illustrations.

A special thank-you to Tommy Farren, former registrar at the Irish Dental Council, and to Paul O'Grady of ThinkMedia for their insightful comments and advice.

I wish also to acknowledge my dear friend and colleague Professor Richard Johns, with whom I worked closely in the Sheffield Institute of Dental Implants. Much of the understanding I gained of the extent of the problems of tooth loss arose out of our close collaboration and his clinical insights during the early pioneer days of dental implants.

Special thanks also to my patients who so readily agreed to allow their photographs to be used and to the many colleagues who supported and believed in this work in the early days when the idea of dental implants was greeted with incredulity.

To those who have given generously of their time and experience and who wish to remain anonymous, you know who you are and I am most grateful to you.

Last but not least, to my family: thank you for all your encouragement with this project and your acceptance of our many lost weekends.

Contents

Foreword by Terry Prone

To lose one tooth is unfortunate. To lose most of them looks like carelessness.

In my case, when it happened, more than twenty-five years ago, it was because my face encountered the steering wheel of my car in the course of a crash which dealt out a number of interesting injuries to me, not least of which was dental destruction. Not that my teeth were anything to write home about but I was used to them. I also earned my living through communications, which does tend to demand that you can speak with relative confidence and be understood with relative ease. The removal of a handful of teeth and their replacement with a partial denture changed all that.

Suddenly I had a lisp. Suddenly I found myself sorting out sentences in advance of giving voice to them, all the better to avoid particular words I knew 'The Partial' wouldn't like. I had grown to think of it in capital letters. The Partial. Hi, I'm Terry Prone and this is The Partial. The Partial had a life and a dance of its own. It had food preferences; forget apples, for starters. I ended up living on couscous. The consequences – anaemia and related horrors – followed, thick and fast.

Now this was in dental implant pre-history. Back then, people didn't casually share with each other the fact that they had one or more dental implants. Nobody knew about dental implants. When they were first mentioned to me, they sounded so prohibitively expensive that only the prospect of receiving compensation for the car crash from the insurance company allowed me even to consider them. But consider them I did. The preliminaries were fun. I got to sit in a little telephone kiosk (remember them?) and have x-rays taken of my dental remnants. Then it got serious. Bone grafts and complications and periods of hiding – all common at that time, when dental implants were in their early stages.

I did, however, meet people in the waiting room who were further along in the process than me and I was encouraged by their experience. In fact, the waiting room had the kind of tone you'd expect of a revivalist meeting in one of the southern states of America. Those who were possessed of dental implants were also possessed of a confidence, an enthusiasm, an urge to proselytise, the like of which I had never previously encountered. Implants, they said, repeatedly, had changed their lives for the better.

Six months later – because it took that long, back then – I was the missionary in the waiting room, explaining to newcomers how miraculous the outcomes were. 'Miraculous' may seem excessive but it was straight reporting. Until I had dental implants, I had a limited understanding of how central one's teeth are to every aspect of life, from health to dealing with people to personal appearance. After dental implants, every week delivered a new awareness of that reality, in the most delightfully positive way.

Hence my willingness – indeed, eagerness – to write this foreword. Because, in the first instance, most of the individuals whose lives could be changed for the better by dental implants are precisely the kind of people who are unlikely to volunteer comments about their current deficits and miseries, so few opportunities present themselves for an implantee to outline just how many benefits this process offers.

Two decades have elapsed since I underwent the surgery. In the intervening years, every aspect of dental implantation has improved. It is simpler. Faster. Cheaper. In the same intervening years, my implants have become a forgotten factor in my life, to be taken for granted.

The science behind implants and their positive place in the history of dental care has never, up to now, been available to non-specialist readers. The gap has now been filled by Professor David Harris, the surgeon who changed my dental life. Even for readers whose every tooth is a wonder of efficacy and strength, his account of this medical breakthrough is fascinating. For those of us who – in the past – didn't bite off more than we could chew, for the simple reason that we could neither bite nor chew – it is an educative encounter with the backdrop to the surgery. For those made miserable by dental problems, it may be a revelation.

Introduction

Have you ever seriously thought about what it might be like to lose all your teeth – every single one of them? Almost certainly not. People who are lucky enough to have all or even some of their natural teeth will be surprised to learn of the severe nature and extent of the problems that can develop following tooth loss. Edentulism is the term used to describe loss of teeth.

I am fully aware that there are many who will view the very notion of describing someone as a 'dental amputee' as an exaggeration, if not a laughable idea. People are naturally kind and sympathetic to problems they can easily observe and empathise with but we all have difficulties relating to health issues that we have not ourselves experienced first hand and cannot easily observe in others. Edentulism falls into this category and the condition is accompanied by the myth that a good set of dentures will solve everything. An important reason this happens is that most people are unaware that loss of all teeth is always followed by a slow and continuing loss of jawbone. This irreversible loss can lead to long-term, severe, physical and functional changes to the facial skeleton.

Although it is reported as being a common nightmare, most people cannot for one moment imagine the extent of the nightmare existence that may lie in wait for many of those who lose all their teeth. Indeed the idea of dentures clacking around in a glass is sometimes seen as a big joke and stories about dentures falling out or being lost as funny stories. For those facing the reality of living with the long-term effects of tooth loss and the changes that emerge over time, it is no laughing matter. This loss can severely affect an individual's appearance, self-confidence, self-esteem and quality of life, as well as their ability to manage a varied and nutritious diet. The World Health Organisation has classified edentulism as a disability. Severe loss of chewing ability can turn patients into oral invalids, in constant pain from ill-fitting dentures, who may manage only a monotonous semi-liquid diet that falls far short of what is necessary to maintain optimum health. This is especially so with the elderly and can even be the cause of sudden death. However, for many people this is just the tip of the iceberg: there is a whole range of underlying disabling and unwanted consequences that may remain hidden beneath the surface, as they are not noticed or appreciated by anyone other than by those who suffer. These include emotional distress and social avoidance as well as problems with relationships and intimacy. The edentulous come to expect little sympathy or understanding for their condition. Their experiences often make them embarrassed and ashamed and they feel they have no option but to suffer in silence.

This book sets out to provide an insight into the difficult condition of edentulism and the modern treatments that are available for it. It is my hope that those who suffer from it will be helped by knowing that the problems that accompany it are not unique to them, that they are not at fault and that modern research has produced effective remedies that are now widely available.

Professor David Harris, December 2014

1

The Dental Amputee:
Dreams, Nightmares and Reality

*Dreams are just reality waiting to happen. Nightmares
are there to say everything is just a dream but nothing is
stopping those dreams from becoming reality.*

Katie Magill

For those who have not lost their teeth, it is understandable that the term 'dental amputee' may sound like an overstatement of the condition. Nothing could be further from the truth. Teeth and the bone that supports them are an essential and, as we will see, a very meaningful body part. Their loss, over time, may have disastrous consequences. Some of those consequences are functional and are easy to imagine, such as an inability to chew foods and enjoy a varied and healthy diet, or difficulties with speech. WHO (2001) classifies edentulousness (loss of all teeth) as a physical impairment.

What is not so obvious is how the loss of all teeth can greatly affect one's quality of life. It is not widely appreciated that becoming edentulous can initiate a cascade of undesirable events that, in turn, affect the functional, emotional, psychological and sexual wellbeing and health of both men and women. The fact that teeth are deeply ingrained in the human psyche can give rise to a wide spectrum of emotional reactions when they are lost, something that may surprise people who still have their teeth. Even dentists can underestimate the full impact of tooth loss on a patient.

Dentists all over Ireland are familiar with some of the more obvious problems faced by dental amputees. They regularly meet patients

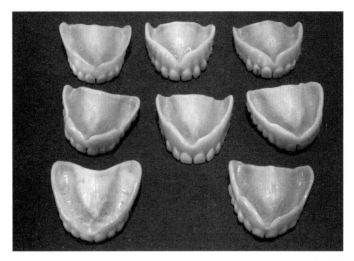

Fig. 1.1

who seek their help. Sometimes, those patients bring with them the evidence of the difficulties they are experiencing. This evidence is, in some cases, housed in a plastic bag. In other cases, it shelters within a clean handkerchief. When either is opened, the dentist sees a set of dentures. Or several sets of dentures (Fig. 1.1).

Ostensibly, the significance of these exhibits is that the patient has never managed to get a properly fitting, comfortable set of dentures. They all work for a while, the patient explains, but then they start to move and rub against the delicate gum tissues, causing soreness and ulceration. The dentist is well aware of the reasons for this and knows that, as a consequence of the loss of all natural teeth, the underlying jawbone structure and shape will inevitably, progressively and irreversibly continue to shrink. The dentures, on the other hand, remain the same as the day they were fitted. Dentures that are perfect this year may be agonising just a few years hence. It's not the fault of dentists or of the companies manufacturing the false teeth. As we will see, it's a consequence of an entirely natural process.

However, complaints about ill-fitting dentures provide little insight into the true extent of the problems of patients. As will become clear in this chapter, there are many reasons why patients are reluctant to disclose the full extent of their problems to their dentist, so they confine themselves to telling them the part of the story they believe will be understood.

Why are they so reluctant to share their problems? Because they believe that anyone who has retained all or most of their teeth cannot, even for a moment, begin to imagine the extent of the emotional, psychological and physical consequences of being toothless. This is not a trivial or unimportant issue but one that, as we will see, goes to the very heart of someone's identity. That's why, in this book, I use the term 'dental amputee'. Nothing less than the word 'amputation' can describe the loss of a vital body part. Furthermore, unlike the loss of other body parts, individuals feel the absence of all their teeth in a uniquely hidden and often personal and shameful way. The fact is that if a person, as a result of an accident, loses any part of their body that is visible they become an immediate object of sympathy. If the loss of the body part results in a serious loss of function they may well be viewed with admiration as they eventually manage to get on with their lives and overcome their handicap. Everyone can easily identify and empathise with that situation. Loss of teeth does not evoke such pity. Nor, in any circumstance, does it evoke admiration.

What is arguably the saddest aspect of this phenomenon is that the patients who come to dental clinics seeking help are in the minority. The majority of dental amputees live with the misery of their condition in silence, in secrecy and with no sense that there is anything they can do about it. They feel very embarrassed about having no teeth of their own and will take great care to try to hide that fact from others. However, in spite of their best efforts, sometimes the problems bubble up in the most unexpected of ways and they suffer greatly when their loss is exposed to others by some chance occurrence or situation.

One patient told me recently that, as she put it, she 'copes by concealing' from herself and everybody else, especially her family, that she wears dentures. This subterfuge broke down when she had to go into hospital for elective surgery and everything changed for the worse. Her condition was brought home to her when a nurse was going through a pre-anaesthetic checklist and asked her if she wore false teeth. She had to admit the truth and the nurse explained that her dentures had to be removed for the duration of her anaesthetic. No matter how kind the nurse was, the patient felt mortified. Theatre nurses will tell you that this is not an uncommon story and that often the first words that such patients utter on recovering from an anaesthetic is a request for the return of their false teeth. She had prepared herself well in advance for the experience of the surgery – which was successful. However, she had not anticipated how upset she would become by the experience of handing over her dentures. She was devastated on being wheeled to the theatre, sans teeth, by a friendly porter who talked to her, and being spoken to by theatre staff and by the surgeon; she was ashamed to respond, lest her lack of teeth be obvious. Even though her teeth were restored to her as soon as she came around from the anaesthetic, the experience changed everything for her. Never again, she decided, would she let herself be so personally diminished by wearing (or in the case of the surgery, not wearing) false teeth. She was clear in her mind that she would have to do something about being edentulous.

Not everybody has a horror story to tell about wearing dentures but many people have. Another woman in her thirties related how she lost her lower dentures when she went swimming. She opened her mouth in the water and they simply floated away. She will forever remember desperately trying to locate them in the sand, repeatedly diving without success. At the same time she was trying to work out how she could get a replacement set of false teeth in a Spanish holiday resort without the other members of the hen party she was with finding out what had happened to her.

People like these two patients often say, 'Do you know, I've never told that to anyone before. You're the first person I've ever told.' That's because loss of teeth is a huge, even a fundamental blow to someone's whole being. People feel lessened by it and even further diminished by the humiliation of the key incident that causes them to seek help. While they may ruefully laugh, having at last told somebody about it, that laugh is partly one of relief that they have, after years of silence, finally revealed the secret about which they feel so ashamed. The yarn never becomes one of those war stories – 'my most embarrassing moment' – that we're normally happy to share with friends and family.

Occasionally, someone's edentulous condition becomes known involuntarily and against their will. One patient was a teacher – senior and highly respected in her school – who, heading down the main staircase one day, opened her mouth to issue a reproof to students engaging in horseplay in the hall below. Her false teeth fell out of her mouth and down the stairs in front of her. It's hard even to imagine how anyone could recover from the loss of dignity resulting from a situation such as this. Anything to do with being edentulous is so embarrassing for the sufferer that not only are they reluctant to talk about it, they find it impossible to be amused by any incident that might have revealed it to others.

Many older people don't see themselves as exceptional in wearing false teeth. Most people under sixty tend to assume that everybody else of their age has their own teeth, so the fact that they wear dentures isolates them and makes them as secretive about it as if they were addicted to some illicit substance. Nobody must ever find out because nobody would understand. Nobody must ever find out because they would inevitably think less of the edentulous person. Nobody must ever find out because the details of their condition so humiliate the person wearing false teeth that, even admitting to them out loud to a third party somehow makes things worse.

When someone who has lost all their teeth hears about the possibilities of dental implants and attends for treatment, they will not, in most cases, initially disclose to the dentist the extent of the problems they are experiencing. A small majority of those seeking help are women and they will usually say that they're having difficulty with their false teeth. A typical interview may go as follows.

'How long have you been wearing dentures?'

'I've been wearing them about twenty years,' they say. 'I would like to see if I could have implants.' They would often prefer not to talk any more about the problems they are having but because it is so important to know what their symptoms and expectations are before any treatment is undertaken, further questions are necessary.

'What exactly are the problems you are having that make you believe implants might help?'

'Oh, well, my teeth are loose and I can't eat properly. My gum gets a bit sore and I'm just always uncomfortable.'

'Well now, if you were able to have dentures that fitted securely and comfortably, so you would be able to chew what you like and they wouldn't let you down, would you…?'

At this point they usually interrupt. 'Oh no, no, no,' they say. 'I want implants!'

So now we know there are some underlying and undisclosed reasons why they are seeking help. What is going on is extremely personal and, since this is their first visit, they may have great difficulty revealing or acknowledging it. It can take a while to elicit the full truth and, sometimes the full truth does not emerge until after the completion of treatment, if at all. On occasion, the information comes indirectly and by accident. One patient got talking to another in the waiting room and enquired if she'd had implants.

'Yes. Best thing that ever happened to me,' was the reply.

'I had them, too,' the other patient said and fell silent.

'Was it not a good experience for you?'

'Oh, it was. It's changed my life.'

Another silence.

'Since I lost all my teeth I hadn't had sex – my husband and I hadn't had sex in fifteen years.

'What?'

'I couldn't bring myself to make love when I had horrible loose false teeth. Taking them out was worse and my husband hated them too.'

This may surprise you but, as we will see in the following chapters, problems with intimacy and libido are not unusual following loss of teeth and this can affect both partners.

The psychological and emotional significance of teeth

This significance can better be appreciated by considering the many important functions associated with the mouth, which is, after all, one of the most intimate and sensitive areas of the human body. These functions include suckling, chewing, taste, drinking, swallowing, breathing, speech and singing, expression of feelings, smiling, laughter, intimacy and sex. They include, in other words, almost all the functions that make us social animals. Is it any wonder that becoming toothless tends to isolate the sufferer?

The early years

The integration of the mouth into our psyche begins at birth. The mouth provides an essential survival role in suckling and comforting and is also the foundation of a most important early bonding and communication process between baby and mother. Who will not crumble at the first smile of a baby?

In their early years, children explore the world by attempting to place almost all the objects they encounter into their mouths. There they are closely examined for texture, shape and taste. This represents an important method by which small children investigate and build up their internal and personal picture of the world. Babies will calm down and be comforted by sucking on soothers or even on their own thumb. Mothers will instinctively kiss an upset child. Parents kiss their children to show them they are loved. Disagreements will often end with children being told to kiss and make up.

The appearance of the baby teeth allows the weaning process to become complete and their subsequent loss is marked in many cultures by the arrival of the tooth fairy. The appearance of the first adult tooth is celebrated and marks a transition in growth.

During teenage years, regular and harmonious white teeth are highly prized as an attractive feature. This is often anticipated by parents and creates a demand for orthodontic treatment in childhood or adolescence to prevent irregularities and overcrowding of the teeth in adult life. Emotional intimacy with another person begins with the first kiss. Expressions of joy, welcome and indeed many more subtle communications are contained within the way we smile. It is worth noting that smiling itself is a uniquely human activity, in spite of what some dog and cat owners will tell you. It is quite a different phenomenon from the pulling back of the lips and baring of teeth seen in chimpanzees and other animals that in fact is nearly always a display of aggression.

The teeth in Penfield's homunculus studies

The importance we instinctively and often unconsciously attach to the mouth, teeth and lips is well illustrated in the homunculus studies that Wilder Penfield, a great Canadian neurosurgeon, carried out in the 1950s. (Homunculus is the Latin word for 'little man'.) Penfield was an innovator who perfected surgical treatment for intractable epilepsy. He was fascinated by the way the brain worked and developed ways to observe the living brain directly in humans and witness how it responded to electrical stimuli. He produced a graphic representation of the surface of the brain showing the extent to which various parts of the body are represented. The result is often called a homunculus.

Penfield set out to investigate the functions of the human cerebral hemispheres, those large areas of the brain that lie immediately beneath the skullbone. There is a left and a right hemisphere and they are significantly more highly developed in humans than in other mammals, both in size and in function. The outer layer of these hemispheres, called the cerebral cortex, is closely associated with the appreciation of sensation from all parts of the body (the sensory cortex) and the control of movement (the motor cortex).

Penfield selectively applied electrodes to small individual areas of the cerebral cortex in patients who were undergoing surgery for conditions such as uncontrollable epilepsy. The subjects were fully conscious and as a result were able to report any sensations they felt. He could also observe whether the stimuli produced any muscle movement. If you feel squeamish about this type of experiment it is important to note that stimulation of the cerebral cortex does not cause any pain to the subject. Hence it was necessary to use only local anaesthesia to ensure numbness in the scalp area and the surface of the skull. From these investigations Penfield was able to map out the particular areas of the motor and sensory cortex that are associated with sensations arising from different parts of the body. His work clearly showed that some body areas had a larger surface representation than others; in other words, that more of our brainpower is devoted to some parts of our bodies than to others – a lot more of our brainpower.

As can be seen in Fig. 1.2, the teeth, lips, mouth and tongue occupy a major proportion of both the sensory and motor parts of the cerebral cortex, as do the hand and thumb, when compared to the proportion occupied by the rest of the body.

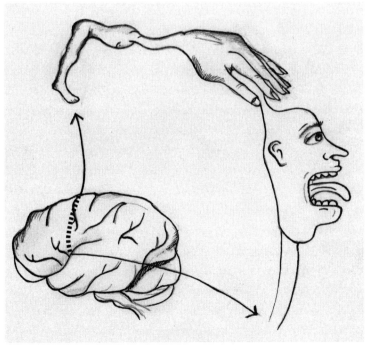

Fig. 1.2
© Professor David Harris: artist Lia Cowan.

Penfield's studies quite elegantly demonstrate the sensitivity and importance of the various roles associated with our teeth and oral structures. They also serve to underline how devastating the loss of functions associated with the mouth and teeth can be. One of those functions is the capacity to smile. From a few weeks after birth, the smile is a central part of how we relate to one another and express joy at the sight of one another. Inevitably, losing your teeth inhibits this most natural component of human body language.

The evolutionary perspective

This brings me to a vitally important point: the embarrassment attached to being without your own teeth is a lot more than wounded vanity. Tooth loss is one of the most vivid intimations of mortality. Even in humans, tooth loss can evoke the evolutionary memory of panic at the threat of death such loss once posed. Animals cannot survive without their teeth. In the wild, loss of teeth is a sentence of death, pure and simple, because the animal can no longer catch, kill or consume its prey. Our subliminal fear of death and the association of toothlessness with getting old reinforce each other. In a society that avoids thinking about death and places a high premium on youth, this can, as we will see in Chapter 2, create a continuing sense of bereavement among people who lose their teeth.

From an evolutionary perspective teeth were essential for survival. A modern soft, cooked diet requires nothing like the chewing ability so essential to our human ancestors, who consumed coarse grains and stripped raw meat and sinews from bones. This kind of diet also necessitated the development of strong jaw muscles. Recovered jaws of primitive man show distinct flattening and wear facets on the teeth, which are characteristic of these activities.

But notably absent from these ancient skulls is evidence of tooth decay or gum disease. These common diseases are entirely associated with the refined carbohydrates in the form of starches and sugars so favoured by a modern diet.

So even though our Stone Age ancestors had a tough time finding and masticating food, for the most part their teeth did not rot from being bathed in sugar.

Human bites

Teeth have even had a function in combat. The expression 'to fight tooth and nail' is used to convey a fight for survival. Human bites are certainly not unknown in cases of assault and are regularly seen in emergency departments. Human bites can be very dangerous, with a high potential to cause infections.

A widely publicised example in sport was the heavyweight boxing fight during which Mike Tyson bit off part of the ear of his opponent, Evander Holyfield, in June 1987. More recently, at the 2014 soccer World Cup in Brazil, the Uruguayan footballer Luis Suarez caused outrage when he bit the shoulder of Italian defender Giorgio Chiellini during a match.

Dreams and tooth loss

The pivotal role of teeth in our psyche is also reflected by the number of people who report dreams or nightmares centred on losing their teeth. A Google search for 'tooth loss and dreams' brings up in excess of half a million entries. It would appear from some of these entries that those who like to interpret dreams report that it is one of the more common nightmares they are asked about. It is certainly one that many patients report and they also say that these dreams are accompanied by most unpleasant feelings, especially feelings of insecurity.

Fear of dentistry

Another indicator of the deep emotional role of teeth is the number of people who avoid attending for dental treatment because of fear of dentistry. This has been estimated to be as much as 50 per cent of the adult population. A proportion of these individuals have developed a true dental phobia. Sometimes this can be traced back to a bad early experience or to one that threatened the passage of air through the nose or mouth, such as a near-drowning incident, or to anything that caused a temporary inability to breathe. But most dental phobics are simply fearful of any intrusion or invasion into this intimate and sensitive area, without being able to identify exactly why. For them, the sight, sounds or smells of a dental surgery can induce an involuntary release of hormones from a part of the brain known as the hypothalamus. This in turn causes a reaction known as the 'fight or flight' reaction.

The fight or flight reaction was first described in the 1920s by a Harvard physiologist, Walter Cannon, and is considered to be an essential survival response in human evolution. It is the response that allowed our ancestors to run like the wind when they sighted a buffalo or a tiger. It is the exact opposite of the relaxation response and is an inappropriately stressful one for a patient in the dental surgery. Very nervous dental patients will be most familiar with the effects of this reaction: a rapid heartbeat, pallor as a result of diversion of bloodflow away from the skin to large muscle groups, a rise in blood pressure and the onset of sweating. Logic and reason are of no help in this situation as the body prepares to fight or flee, not relax. In the most difficult cases people find they cannot bring themselves to attend for treatment unless forced to by the onset of extreme pain or swelling. Even people who might be considered extraordinarily brave in their daily activities or hobbies, such as skydivers, mountaineers, rugby players or even tough special forces personnel are capable of turning to jelly at the thought of having to go to the dentist.

This emotional and psychological aspect of teeth was used to great effect in the film *Marathon Man*, in which Laurence Olivier appeared as the sadistic inquisitor of a helpless and restrained Dustin Hoffman. The torture involved drilling into his live teeth. This film probably set attendance at dentists' surgeries back for years. Anyone who has seen it will tell you how horrific this particular scene was although, if you look closely, you will see that the director does not show any graphic details. All the viewer hears is the sound of the drill while they see a movement towards the mouth. That's it. That's all. The director, knowing how people react to dentistry (even with an anaesthetic), anticipated correctly that he could leave it entirely to the imagination of the audience to fill in any grim horrors they themselves might care to conjure up.

The availability of modern sedative agents, together with a greater understanding of the problem by dentists, can enable nervous patients to undergo dental care without stress.

People who lose a limb as a result of an accident or through surgery often complain of an odd and distressing condition known as 'phantom limb' pain. For example, although they know that they no longer have a left leg below the knee, some part of their brain tells them that a part of the missing limb is still present and hurting. People who lose all their teeth may not suffer any great physical pain but they can suffer enormous emotional and psychological pain and suffer it in isolation.

The contrast between the isolation felt by the edentulous and the external perception of toothlessness is sharp and, for the toothless patient, painful. Wearing dentures is often reduced to the joke of 'granny's teeth in the glass by the bedside' and many joke shops sell miniature spring-loaded clacking teeth. For years, postcards involving crude cartoons of false teeth were a staple in the souvenir shops of British seaside resorts. The assumption was that it was all a joke. Those creating the cheap laugh probably never realised how very cruel this joke was for the people involved.

2

Emotional and Psychological Effects of Tooth Loss

Last scene of all,
That ends this strange eventful history,
Is second childishness and mere oblivion,
Sans teeth, sans eyes, sans taste, sans everything.

William Shakespeare, *As You Like It*

Edentulism is a life sentence. As we will see, it can actually shorten your life. It is also very much associated with old age, loss of faculties, powerlessness and general physical and mental decline. Shakespeare eloquently sums this up at the end of the soliloquy spoken by the melancholy Jaccques in *As You Like It* (beginning 'All the world's a stage…').

A study, 'The Emotional Effects of Tooth Loss in Edentulous People', undertaken by a team led by Dr J. Fiske and published in the *British Dental Journal* in 1998, provides a rare scientific insight into the wide range of emotional and psychological effects of tooth loss in an older population. Participants enrolled in this study had a mean age of seventy and had been toothless, on average, for eighteen years. Their reactions to and feelings about tooth loss are explored in detail. The findings will surprise many people and are worth considering in some detail. The study found that tooth loss can be both disabling and a handicap. It can have a profound effect on the lives of some people, even those who are apparently coping well with dentures. The paper concludes that the dental profession itself needs to consider how it can prepare people better for the effects of tooth loss.

Five important themes emerge from this study:

- Bereavement
- Acceptance, Adaptation and Disability
- Self-confidence and self-esteem
- Changes in appearance and self-image
- Taboo, secrecy and privacy

The exploration of these themes provides a valuable insight into the extent to which patients can be adversely affected: it matches my own experience in helping edentulous patients over the past thirty years.

Bereavement (and the five stages of grief)

The study found that a sense of bereavement is not uncommon as an initial response, especially when the loss occurs suddenly as a result of a traumatic accident or an underlying disease of which the patient may have been unaware. Patients truly mourn their loss and will go through the full gamut of the five stages of grief that psychiatrist Elisabeth Kübler-Ross originally described in her 1969 book, *On Death and Dying:*

1. Denial: 'This can't be happening to me.'
2. Anger: 'Why is this happening? Who is to blame?'
3. Bargaining: 'Make this not happen and in return I will...'
4. Depression: 'I'm too sad to do anything.'
5. Acceptance: 'I'm at peace with what happened.'

At first a patient may refuse to believe that there is any problem at all. This initial denial is gradually replaced by a realisation that an irreversible loss and disability have occurred. The realisation sometimes takes place only when the individual has realised the inadequacy and consequences of the wearing of dentures, things that tends to become more obvious over time.

After this the patient may become very angry and look for someone to blame. This anger may initially be directed against the dentist who removed the teeth, or against the person who caused the accident but, more often, a patient's anger is directed against him or herself. Patients can conclude, quite unjustifiably, that they are the authors of their own misfortune. They may feel ashamed of neglecting their dental care or bitterly regret that they did not look after their teeth better. They do not realise that the feelings they are experiencing are common and soon become convinced that they are the only ones who feel this way. Of course extreme neglect can be a cause of tooth loss but often the reasons are more complex. Although tooth decay (dental caries) is a major cause of tooth loss, more often than not gum disease that remains undetected or untreated is the main cause in adults.

How can such disease remain undetected? Because it takes places unseen beneath the gum tissues and the early signs may be no more than bleeding that occurs on brushing. Bleeding in this way is never normal: it is an early warning sign and requires professional attention. The problem is that as the disease progresses deeper beneath the gums, the bleeding may stop. The patient may now think the problem has gone away. However, the reality is that this sometimes marks a phase when a quiet, painless and progressive destruction of the bone that supports the teeth has begun. There are few things in dentistry more upsetting than to have tell a patient, with a perfect set of teeth and who has never needed a filling in their life, that they will now lose them all as result of undetected gum disease. It is especially sad because, with rare exceptions, those teeth could have been saved with early corrective and preventive treatment. In this respect the care provided by dental hygienists is particularly important.

Patients may indulge in a process of mental bargaining but find out that in reality the tooth fairy comes around only once and to small children.

Those who cannot function well with dentures can go through a stage of severe depression and withdrawal that may affect all aspects of their lives.

Acceptance, adaptation and disability

Eventually, if no other solution is offered to them, those who have lost their teeth may gradually and reluctantly learn to accept the situation and get on with their lives. Their ability to do this successfully will depend on the extent of their problems, their own outlook and expectations for their quality of life and their physical ability to cope with dentures. As we will see, even if patients manage well with dentures at first, the situation is not stable. Dentures become more problematic over time because of the long-term changes that occur in the jawbone, which, sadly, are irreversible.

The acceptance stage involves coming to terms with any disabilities that are experienced as a result of tooth loss. All those affected find that they change their behaviour in some way in an effort to adapt to this new reality. Such changes may be very subtle. They may be unconsciously introduced and the person themselves may remain unaware that they have occurred. For example, a person who has lost all their teeth sometimes alters their diet without fully realising that they're afraid to choose certain foods they cannot comfortably manage. Others may adopt more major changes that will impact heavily on their quality of life, for example giving up playing a wind instrument or avoiding eating in restaurants or going to business dinners. A host of variable factors will determine the extent to which such changes occur. Age, general and specific health conditions, work, personality, lifestyle and expectations, social interactions in general as well as the length of time since the teeth have been lost – all these elements play a role. Such a wide variety of reactions is not surprising given people's diverse personalities and lifestyles.

Self-confidence and self-esteem

In Fiske's study, many patients report a loss of self-confidence and self-esteem as a result of losing their teeth. This loss may be extreme and may adversely affect social activities and successful interaction with others. For teenagers and young adults it can be exceptionally severe, especially if they have been conscientiously looking after their oral hygiene and dental care and then lose their teeth as a result of a traumatic accident or a medical condition.

An example is the rare condition of juvenile periodontitis, which results in patients losing all their teeth at a young age despite intensive treatment. Such loss, which is totally beyond their control, can leave them feeling less than a whole person and dramatically different from their peers. Young people often say, 'Someone of my age should not have to wear dentures.' They do not want anyone to know they are wearing dentures and will go to great lengths to try and disguise the fact. They often avoid activities and situations that might draw attention to their problem: for example, covering their mouth with their hand when they laugh or smile or learning to restrict the movement of their lips. Sports activities become a nightmare for them. Even swimming represents a threat, as dentures can easily float out of the mouth. During the sensitive teenage years, when a spot on the chin can be considered a major disaster, tooth loss and dentures are dreadfully hard to accept and adapt to.

These feelings are not confined to younger people: mature adults often report similar reactions.

Relationships and intimacy

Relationships and intimacy can also become a major issue, as a result of deep-rooted feelings in the patient or in the dentate partner. I have met several patients who were not able to enjoy a sexual relationship because one of the partners wore dentures. In one couple, this avoidance of sex had left them childless. Intimacy problems are probably more common than realised, as patients are understandably reluctant to talk about this most personal of matters. Often they do not mention them until after they have been successfully rehabilitated by means of dental implants and have developed an understanding and trusting relationship with their dentist. Men and women alike reported to Fiske's investigators that their libido was adversely affected. The association of teeth with youth and vitality and the loss of them with powerlessness, ageing and decay probably underlies many of these feelings. If a woman's loss of teeth coincides with the onset of menopause, the emotional effects are likely to be more severe.

A lot more could be written about this. A lot more should have been written about it. But even in the frankest films, books and TV series, edentulousness does not figure. It is the ultimate embarrassment, the ultimate relationship-destroying disability. It has never, to my knowledge, featured in *Sex and the City*.

Changes in appearance and self-image

Over the years an individual's appearance can change dramatically as a result of wearing full dentures. Although some dentures can initially look extremely good and function reasonably well, a variety of adverse changes to appearance, as well as the loss of chewing ability, can occur over time. These changes and the reasons they occur are discussed in detail in Chapter 3. The end result may be premature ageing of the face and a greatly diminished ability to chew food and enjoy a varied diet.

An additional factor is that, because of ongoing long-term changes in the shape of the mouth, dentures can become loose and difficult to retain. This has given rise to a worldwide industry that makes and sells denture adhesives. I have yet to meet a patient who is content with having to use these gooey pastes or powders in their mouth. Most do so only out of desperation – sometimes with unexpected and disastrous results. Some of these products have recently been withdrawn from the market because of the discovery of dangerous side-effects in some people who used them. The adhesives involved all contained the mineral zinc. Excessive absorption of zinc from the adhesives placed beneath the denture caused severe neurological damage in some patients. It may not generally be realised that chemicals substances can enter into the bloodstream through the tissues of the mouth – it is an excellent location for the quick absorption of chemicals and drugs. Pharmaceutical companies produce many drugs, for example medicines to reduce blood pressure or dilate coronary vessels in acute angina, in a formulation that can be placed beneath the tongue to ensure rapid absorption and effect. In the case of denture adhesives containing zinc – a substance that is beneficial to health in small doses – the amount being absorbed was so great that it amounted to a toxic overdose. The manufacturers claimed that this occurred only because people were using the product in much larger quantities and more frequently than recommended. I believe that this may well be the case, surely a testimony to the desperate attempts some denture wearers make to overcome the extreme difficulties they encounter and the failure of the adhesive to solve their denture problems when used as recommended. More recently zinc has become a less common component of dental adhesives.

When they start having problems with their dentures, denture-wearers often change their behaviour. Eating out can become a nightmare. Patients report that when they go to a restaurant and look at a menu it is to see what they can manage to eat rather than what would be nice to eat. Having full upper dentures covering the palate changes the taste of food. The peppermint flavour of some retaining adhesives further confuses the taste buds. Eating out, for many denture-wearers, becomes so joyless that many avoid the embarrassment simply by refusing invitations.

Taboo, secrecy and privacy

Denture wearers can feel desperately isolated with their problems. This feeling of isolation may arise from their being ashamed of their condition or from feelings of guilt that they may have been the cause of it. They may also feel guilty that they are unable to cope with dentures in a way that they imagine others must be able to do. They are fearful that they may be laughed at and that no one will understand their problems, so they are really surprised to hear that they are not alone. Even when they have physical pain from denture wearing, they are reluctant to complain. They may not feel that they deserve the painful ulcers on their gums that distract them throughout the day but they anticipate that they will receive little sympathy from others. A black eye or back pain can be empathised with much more easily. Their situation is further complicated by the belief that dentists prefer to do interesting work saving teeth and regard someone who has lost all their teeth as a failure. The former has an element of truth in it: the latter doesn't. When they encounter a patient with two or three sets of dentures hidden in a clean, crumpled handkerchief, many dentists experience the sinking feeling that whatever solution they come up with may not serve the patient for very long.

All this results in a great deal of secrecy developing around the issue. 'My partner or children have never seen me without my teeth so they don't know I have no teeth,' patients presenting for dental implants often say.

Two quotations from Fiske's study illustrate the extent of the secrecy and embarrassment surrounding the loss of teeth:

'I could have spoken openly about the death of a friend but not the death of my teeth.'

'No, I don't think people did [discuss tooth loss]. It's like that word "cancer", isn't it?'

When patients present for treatment and find they are talking to a sympathetic person who understands their problems and can help them, they may experience an emotional release. They can find it difficult to talk about it without sobbing or their eyes welling up because it is the first time they have been able to talk openly about it. Over the years many of my implant patients have counselled others who are about to undergo treatment and this recognition of shared suffering has sometimes led to enduring friendships.

Very extensive emotional and psychological disability can arise from tooth loss. Some 45 per cent of those interviewed for Fiske's study stated that they felt that they had been inadequately prepared for the problems that faced them. They accepted that in some cases the dentist might have offered an explanation but they were probably too anxious at the time to take it on board. It was clear from the study that we dentists need to do a better job in this area. Patients need time to absorb information and consider the consequences of tooth loss prior to the appointment at which the teeth are to be removed. This information needs to be delivered in a clear and sympathetic fashion.

Over the years I have had several patients who were diagnosed with cancer either before or during implant treatment. Some of these, who underwent extensive surgery and chemotherapy, said to me, 'I can deal with the cancer but not with the dentures.'

Perhaps the extent to which tooth loss can affect a person is best exemplified by the quintessential case of a patient who saw moving beyond toothlessness almost as a matter of life and death. This happened in my own clinic about twenty years ago when a lady who hated being without her teeth and wearing dentures decided to have them replaced by implants. She was scheduled for treatment and then cancelled her appointment. Or rather she postponed the treatment day but did not reschedule. In fact, she effectively disappeared. We lost contact with her for almost two years. Then, out of the blue, she returned. A treatment was arranged and this time she went ahead. When it was completed she was delighted with the results.

Only at this point – on completion of her treatment – did she reveal the reason for her two-year absence. It happened that at the time her dental surgery was originally scheduled, she had unexpectedly been diagnosed with cancer. Her immediate priority was to undergo the necessary treatment for her illness. This involved both surgery and chemotherapy and she was told that she had perhaps at best three to five years to live. She was convinced that, if I became aware of this prognosis, I would not have provided her with dental implants. It was this fear that caused her to disappear and to return only when the signs of her illness were no longer obvious. She was not in denial. She knew she was going to die but, as she subsequently told me, she had decided that, whatever her future, she did not want to go to her grave with dentures.

In fact, she survived for almost eight years after her treatment and, in spite of her illness and the accompanying prognosis, she told me that the decision she had made to go ahead with the implants had given her final years a dignity they would otherwise have lacked.

Physical and Functional Changes that Result from Tooth Loss

Them bones, them bones

The previous chapter dealt with the psychological and emotional effects of tooth loss. It also alluded to the physical and functional changes that occur which are so distressing for patients. These problems arise directly as a result of the way the jawbone changes shape and structure following the loss of teeth. Patients often describe this as 'gum shrinkage', whereas, in fact, it is actually the jawbone that 'shrinks'. To explain these physical changes more fully I will try to provide some insight into the extraordinary and miraculous nature of bone.

The majority of people without a background in biology probably think of bone as being a fixed, solid and unchanging entity, something like solid ivory. Nothing could be further from the truth. If bone were made of solid ivory we would simply collapse under the weight of our skeletons. Bone is constantly changing its structure and form, twenty-four hours a day, seven days a week – and this includes the jawbones. The way this is achieved is an intriguing story and a perfect example of how Mother Nature acts with the greatest economy to provide the most beneficial outcome at the lowest biological cost.

Everybody understands that the bony skeleton is something that develops its shape and size as it grows continually throughout childhood and adolescence. It is somewhat less obvious that a similar mechanism is at work in adults. Here it is necessary to get a little technical. Bone is always in a state of change as it alters its form and shape in response to the demands that are placed on it. Hence it creates denser and stronger bone in the direction in which most stress is placed on it. This feature allows the body to provide a structure to bone that ensures that it is strongest where it needs to be strong and kept lighter and less dense where strength is not normally required. For example the bones in our legs become structured in a way that provides greatest strength in a vertical direction. This arrangement allows us to jump, run, walk and carry our body weight without the danger of their breaking. The mechanism does, however, make it easier for a break to occur when they receive a blow from the side.

Our skeletal structure has evolved over many millennia since the first animals developed a primitive skeleton. Within our bone, a carefully orchestrated balancing act is constantly at work, whereby special cells (osteoclasts) are continually breaking down older bone, while other cells (osteoblasts) are continually repairing and forming new bone. This phenomenon is known as bone resorbtion and bone deposition. In healthy fully-grown adults the amount of bone formed and the amount of bone removed must more or less balance out. This balance is maintained under the influence of a wide variety of growth hormones, the sex hormones oestrogen and progesterone, testosterone, thyroid and parathyroid hormones and vitamin D – all of which are produced, secreted and carefully controlled within the body. Startling as it may seem, we will all replace our entire skeleton on a regular basis during our lifetime.

Osteoporosis

Should the balance shift towards bone loss in adults, osteoporosis will result and calcium is withdrawn from bone, which becomes less dense. In extreme cases spontaneous bone fractures can occur. Women, who undergo many hormonal changes around menopause, have a much greater risk than men of developing osteoporosis, with associated changes in both volume and density of the bone. However, men are not immune to osteoporosis. Because of the extent of this condition in the ageing population treatment is very much aimed at prevention and includes exercise, ensuring a healthy diet with adequate amounts of calcium, dietary supplements and sometimes the use of specific drugs. It is also helpful to avoid smoking and excessive alcohol and caffeine intake.

The shift towards bone deposition is normal in growing children, when the bony skeleton is enlarging, and also during the growth spurts seen in adolescents. But if the balance shifts towards excess bone deposition in adults, it is always the result of disease processes (such as acromegaly, a serious condition resulting from an excess of growth hormone).

One of the most potentially devastating consequences of losing one's teeth is the bone loss that follows. This change is a natural function of the body and not a disease. The well known phrase, 'If you don't use it, you lose it,' really applies to bone. This is the reason that exercise is recommended to help to prevent osteoporosis. Unlike most mechanical things that wear out from overuse, the main obstacle to successfully maintaining strong healthy bones is underuse. Walking and other weight-bearing exercises stimulate bone by the action of the muscles that are attached and by direct application of weight. This stimulation is known technically as 'loading' bone. It is well documented that such loading is absolutely necessary if the body is to be stimulated into bone-production rather than bone-loss mode. The opposite will occur in the absence of loading. An interesting example is the way in which the lack of gravity and weightlessness, experienced in outer space, poses problems for those who spend prolonged periods on the orbiting international space station. Because the weightlessness experienced reduces the stimulus to the bony skeleton, significant bone loss can result. This is the reason astronauts undergo a regular exercise programme whilst in orbit to try to maintain normal bone deposition.

In the case of the jawbones, it is the presence of functioning teeth that provides the necessary load to maintain bone. When a significant number of teeth have been removed there is an initial loss of the bone that made up the teeth sockets – so-called alveolar bone. This loss usually occurs relatively quickly over a three-month period. This is

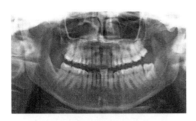

Fig. 3.1

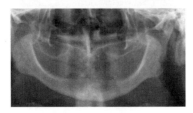

Fig. 3.2

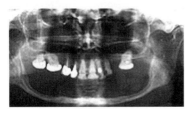

Fig. 3.3

followed by a much slower but continual and irreversible loss of the main body of the jawbone, a loss that will continue over a patient's lifetime, producing devastating changes in both function and appearance.

Fig. 3.1 shows an x-ray of a patient with upper and lower teeth present. X-rays always cast dark shadows and the denser the structures within the jaws the less easy it is for x-rays to pass through. Any fillings present show up as white as the metal in them totally blocks the passage of x-rays. The teeth are more dense than bone and therefore appear less dark and show up more clearly. The grey area around the teeth and below is bone; this bone around the roots of the teeth is known as alveolar bone.

Fig. 3.2 shows the situation when all teeth have been lost. It can be seen that the alveolar bone is no longer present.

Fig. 3.3 shows what can happen after many years when the on-going bone loss has further reduced the remaining volume of bone.

A comparison of Fig. 3.2 and Fig. 3.3 illustrates the degree of bone loss that has occurred over time. This progressive bone loss is also shown in the sequence in Fig. 3.4, from which it is obvious that the final outcome is a thin and fragile jawbone.

The role of the teeth in the development of the jaw is also seen in the fortunately rare hereditary condition of ectodermal dysplasia. In this condition teeth entirely fail to develop. The jawbones of children affected by the condition will not develop normally due to the lack of the stimulus usually provided by teeth. The result is that the jawbones remain small, with no tooth-bearing area, which causes a sunken and aged appearance in childhood.

Traditionally, when adults lose all their teeth, dentures, known as complete removable dentures, replace them. One of the most disappointing aspects of wearing complete dentures is that they do not appear to provide the necessary pressure to the underlying bone for it to maintain its normal structure. It is as if the gum tissues themselves absorb the eating forces placed on dentures and fail to transmit these to the underlying bone, with the result that it will shrink and recede

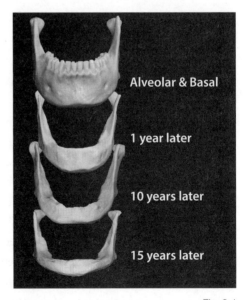

Fig. 3.4
© *Paul Harris.*

over time. Complete dentures are therefore only a temporary solution to a deteriorating problem.

The denture sinks into the receding tissues, becomes loose and unstable and may begin to impinge on the delicate soft tissue of the mouth, causing ulcers and pain. In advanced cases, nerves, which originally lay deep within the body of the bone, become superficial and lie just beneath the gum tissues. They may then become trapped under the denture and cause severe pain.

In extreme cases, the bone can become so thin and fragile that the lower jaw may simply fracture in the same way that hip and spinal fractures can occur as a result of osteoporosis. Such a spontaneous fracture, which is fortunately rare, can occur as a result of quite small chewing pressures.

In the early stages of denture wearing, problems can be initially dealt with by a 'reline' of the denture, in which the existing denture is altered in the laboratory to fit the new shape in the mouth. At some stage it will probably be necessary to fit new dentures to try to improve function, comfort and appearance. This new denture will, necessarily, be bigger and bulkier than the original as it has to replace the tissues that have been lost. Over time this ongoing loss of jawbone will result in lack of adequate support for a bulky denture. At this stage patients may find that they cannot manage with it at all – even when using lots of denture adhesives.

Prior to the availability of osseointegrated dental implants, many surgical procedures were carried out to try to compensate for these deleterious effects. These included taking bone from another part of the body, such as the hip and placing (grafting) it on to the jaw in an attempt to build it up again. Such approaches were found to be ineffective. Bone grafts initially worked well but it was quickly discovered that they suffered the same fate as the original bone. In the absence of sufficient pressure to stimulate the bone, it was simply reabsorbed by the body over a relatively short period of time. Before the availability of implants, careful dental practitioners went to great lengths to retain and treat even a few roots of teeth when they made complete dentures. They recognised that these retained roots could serve an important function. Lying underneath the dentures, the roots transmitted the denture loads directly into the bone. The stimulus that resulted was sufficient to delay the onset and extent of bone loss. (The roots were treated to ensure that no infection was associated with them, as this would cause further bone loss.)

It was not until the pioneering research work carried out by Professor Brånemark (described in Chapter 7) that it became clear that implants could prevent this bone loss occurring over long periods after all teeth have been lost.

Of course jawbone can be lost for other reasons. Facial trauma, for example as a result of road traffic accidents or even severe sporting injuries, can leave a patient with difficulties in coping with any type of denture.

Congenital abnormalities such as cleft palate can cause many problems. This condition can result in a large or complete defect of the palate, leaving an opening between the mouth and the nasal passages. Untreated, this brings about severe functional difficulties when eating, drinking or speaking, as well as causing the teeth to erupt very irregularly.

In most western European countries, including Ireland, there is a national programme that provides excellent care for the treatment of cleft lip and palate. The surgery involved effectively repairs the defects, sometimes with a series of operations commencing in childhood, and is supported by dental treatment and speech therapy. However, every now and again I have come across adult patients with severe clefts who were born before these programmes became available. For the more severely affected, undergoing surgery as an adult proved to be extremely challenging and sometimes the results were disappointing. Many of these patients then had to cope with large dentures, which incorporated a plastic extension (obturator) that blocked up the hole in the palate. The availability of implants, which could act as anchors for denture retention and support, was extremely helpful to them.

Distressing loss of bone can also result when major surgery is required to treat oral and facial cancer – especially when it occurs in young people. As we will see, implants can provide many benefits for the rehabilitation of such patients.

The changes in bone structure that have been described mean that a complete denture can be considered only a temporary solution to a continually deteriorating situation. Throughout the world, life expectancy is on a significant upward trend. As people are living longer, wearing dentures over the long term can have a serious impact on their ability to function satisfactorily, as well as their ability to chew and maintain a nutritious and varied diet. This will adversely affect their quality of life.

4

Never Say Die:
The Ageing Time Bomb

Grow old along with me!
The best is yet to be.
The last of life, for which the first was made…
Robert Browning (1812-89)

These lines by Robert Browning have enthralled lovers since the moment his quill hit the paper. He wrote them for his adored poet wife, Elizabeth Barrett Browning, and – although he surely knew that she had been a drug addict since she was in her twenties and continued to be addicted to morphine, in the form of laudanum, throughout their marriage – Browning probably did hope that they would grow old together.

It was not to be. Elizabeth, born in 1806, died in 1861, when she was just fifty-five. Her husband was to outlive her by nearly three decades. However, given life expectancy during the 19th century, the chances were tiny that the couple would grow old together in the way we in the twenty-first century might imagine it.

People simply didn't live as long, two hundred years ago, as they do today. Many children died at birth. Throughout life, infections like tuberculosis decimated the population. Poor housing and inadequate nutrition shortened the lives of the poor. Chancellor Otto von Bismarck's introduction of the old-age pension in Germany in 1888 was a major step forward. For the first time, people over sixty-five would receive annuity payments from the state. This was not, however, likely to bankrupt the national treasury: the average life expectancy at the time was forty-five and many would not live long enough to collect.

We have no idea how long anyone might have expected to live in most of the centuries of history because no records were kept. We know that a large number of children never survived to become teenagers and that the nobility tended to live longer than the poor. We also know that diseases such as bubonic plaque, smallpox and diphtheria culled members of the rich and poor classes alike. It was only during the 19th century that records for national populations first became available in six European countries. In 1804 life expectancy in Europe was forty-one; by 1900, it had risen by almost a decade to just over fifty years. Another ten-year gain was registered by 1930 and by 1960 life expectancy had reached seventy-two and women lived longer than men.

Today we are witnessing a major change in the age structure of populations throughout the world. Put simply, there is a global trend that future generations of people are going to live longer – much longer. With lower birth rates and falling fertility rates worldwide this increase of elderly people in the population is being accompanied by a decrease in younger members. In Ireland and the UK we have reached the point that, for the first time, our population has a greater number of people over the age of sixty-five than those under the age of five. This transition raises many practical issues and is bringing about a sea change in how our society perceives the role of the ageing population. It represents a major achievement in public health but it is a truly monumental change in our society and poses great economic, health and care challenges for our future.

One of the immediate consequences of the increase in our greying society is that throughout Europe governments are now faced with the prospect of providing pensions for much longer periods. This is the reason that many of them are seeking to raise the age at which we start receiving our pensions.

What population changes can we expect in Ireland? The 2006 National Census for Ireland showed that approximately 470,000 people were over the age of sixty-five and 24 per cent of these were over the age of eighty. Projections from the Central Statistics Office indicate that these numbers are set to increase significantly. By 2036 the numbers of those over sixty-five will exceed 1.1 million. But by far the greatest increase will be in those over eighty years of age, who are expected to number 323,000.

By 2030 it is expected that the proportion of the population aged over sixty-five will increase by 100 per cent, those over eighty-five by 150 per cent and – wait for it – with a 400 per cent increase in those over a hundred years old.

There are many reasons why we have seen this dramatic increase in longevity since the 19th century. Initially it was certainly due to the improvement in living conditions and the availability of clean water and sewage. These changes were accompanied by significant advances in medical care, such as the development of vaccines and antibiotics. With improved social and economic conditions, public health measures and better nutrition, we have seen many of the killer diseases, such as scarlet fever, measles, tuberculosis, polio and smallpox being virtually eliminated. In more recent years a better understanding of the benefits of a healthy lifestyle is having an important impact.

Living longer can produce its own problems if it is accompanied by the onset of disease and disability. The many conditions that we are more likely to face as we get older include dementia, stroke, heart disease, cancer, diabetes, depression, osteoporosis and arthritis. In recent years perhaps the most publicised has been Alzheimer's disease, a type of dementia that robs people of their independence and their capacity to understand or relate to the world around them.

Yes, of course, we all would like to live longer but would we really want to do so if it meant physical incapacity, mental impairment and loss of dignity, disease and high dependency.

There is a growing recognition that a most important challenge is to ensure that, as well as living longer, our quality of life is maintained. We should be able to extend the number of years we can remain healthy and free of disabilities and lead independent lives. The good news is that we now know that many of the common diseases associated with ageing can be prevented, modified or delayed. This is not just a matter of medical advances but greatly influenced by the lifestyle choices we make. For example, a lifestyle that includes moderate intake of alcohol, exercise and good nutrition, as well as an avoidance of smoking, can reduce and favourably modify all these diseases. Early detection of high blood pressure and appropriate medication will significantly reduce the incidence of stroke, heart disease and dementia. Opportunities for social interaction and friendships within communities provide many important benefits for our longevity and quality of life.

We also need to redefine what we mean by 'old'. Older people have traditionally been categorised as those who are over the age of sixty-five – mostly, I guess, by people in their forties – and, until recently, this age was cemented into national legislation in relation to retirement and pensions.

It is ridiculous to suggest that a magic switch is tripped when you reach sixty-five and that you are then over the hill. This artificial age barrier does not take into account the great variation in the resilience, capacities and attitudes of people as they become older. It is now well recognised that chronological age does not always correspond to biological age. It is a much more dynamic process than that. We have all come across the person who is 'old' at sixty and the sprightly ninety-year-old who lives independently and enjoys a good quality of life. Clearly genetics and the onset of disease play a large role in ageing. Many of those who have reached sixty-five realise that life has not ended. Some can look forward to the prospect of deciding how to spend the next twenty years or more, in what has become known as the 'third age'. Families may be reared and career prospects no longer an imperative but third agers want to enjoy a high quality of life, one that is personally satisfying as well as socially useful.

Some developed countries are well on their way to their goal of ensuring that living longer is accompanied by a high quality of life – others not so. Sweden is a good example of this. Currently Swedish men who are sixty-five years of age can expect to live for a further eighteen years, during which 75 per cent can expect a healthy life, and women a further twenty-one years. Healthy life expectancy is significantly lower in Russia and in many eastern European countries who recently joined the EU. Clearly there is much work to be done.

Here in Ireland a key contribution to our understanding the needs of our ageing population is being provided by a major, comprehensive study on all aspects of the ageing process. The Irish LongituDinal Study on Ageing, known as TILDA, is led by principal researcher, Professor Rose Anne Kenny, in Trinity College Dublin. This detailed and innovative study followed 8175 people living in Ireland who were over the age of fifty at the time they agreed to participate. Participants were chosen at random and records taken of many aspects of their health, social life, quality of life and economic circumstances. Although Ireland was slow, in international terms, to carry out this type of study, TILDA is unique in its breadth of study of physical, mental health, social and cognitive measures.

Unlike many other major European studies, which are based on a system of self-reporting using questionnaires, TILDA researchers visit each of the participants in their homes at two-yearly intervals to assess their individual status. Participants are also invited to attend a centre, where their physical, mental and health status are recorded. The study, whilst maintaining its own unique features, has been carefully designed to allow integration of its findings into data gathered from other international studies. The longitudinal aspect of the study means that all the participants are followed up on a regular basis over an initial ten-year period, giving an insight into how well individual ageing progresses over time, rather than taking a 'snapshot' at one particular moment. The results of phase one of the study, published in 2009, have already provided new and significant information. The emerging data will inform the goal of extending the number of healthy, quality years the ageing population can expect to enjoy, as well as future public health policy decisions. Phase two was completed in 2012 and Phase 3 will continue observing this group over a further ten years. Full details, background and status of the TILDA project can be found on the website http://www.tcd.ie/tilda.

Growing old without teeth

Losing all your teeth is possibly the least publicised problem associated with getting older. Dr Alex Comfort's ground breaking book, *Ageing: the Biology of Senescence,* published in 1964, makes no mention whatsoever about dental health.

In contrast to the extensive research and policy formulation in general aspects of the ageing process, very little attention has been paid to dental and oral health and its role in improving both general health and quality of life. However this is rapidly changing. An editorial in *The Lancet* in January 2009 drew attention to the risk factors shared by general health and oral disease and the critical need for prevention of oral disease. The World Health Organisation's bulletin of 2005 also drew attention to the lack of research into the oral health needs of elderly people and their impact on quality of life and stressed the need to develop effective and affordable strategies in this area. The first two waves of the TILDA study did not include any measurements of oral health but is hoped that the third part will include measurement of the oral status of participants in association with a team from Trinity College Dublin Dental School led by Professor Brian O'Connell.

A major step forward was the World Health Organisation publication of an international classification of functioning, disability and health in 2001. In this comprehensive and authoritative document, WHO classified the loss of function and disability produced by tooth loss as a physical impairment. This was a clear and overdue recognition that the loss of all teeth can result in a serious functional deficit. It was the first time that such a prestigious global authority recognised toothlessness as more than a footnote in human life. By classifying it as a physical impairment, WHO implicitly registered not only the psychosocial misery the condition inflicts on millions of people but the fact that it can limit an individual's ability to chew, thereby limiting their diet. Once someone has begun to play safe with food, avoiding meat, al dente vegetables and Granny Smith apples, their nutrition levels drop. I had one patient who lost her teeth in her fifties. Greatly hampered by false teeth, she reduced her diet to white bread (because multi-grain breads caused her such severe problems) mashed potato and couscous. After a few years of this, she ended up with severe anaemia and a range of related health problems, as she wasn't ingesting enough of the nutrients necessary to live a healthy life.

Once it occurs, toothlessness is a disability that does not lessen over time: the opposite is the case as function deteriorates hand-in-hand with the progressive and irreversible shrinkage of the jawbone. What this means, in practical terms, is that the younger you are when you lose all your teeth and the longer you live, the more severe the problems you will encounter. As the condition worsens, it is accompanied by an increasing inability to chew foods properly or even to do so at all without pain. The inevitable outcome is that the choice of foods becomes restricted and only the softest, or semi-liquid ones, are selected. This is especially the case for those living in institutions and it has significant health implications as well as affecting the quality of life enjoyed by older people.

A study of the nutritional status of edentulous patients in Cork Dental School and Hospital carried out by Professor Finbar Allen in 2005 showed that 70 per cent of patients had changed their diet because of dental problems and that this represented a medium risk for the adequacy of their nutrition.

Tooth loss, sudden death and the 'café coronary' syndrome

The inability to chew food properly and the wearing of dentures can cause a threat to your life, especially if you are elderly. In 2011, *The Irish Times* published a report of statements by a coroner in Castlebar, County Mayo, after the death of an elderly person (Fig. 4.1). This gives a real life account of the 'café coronary' syndrome.

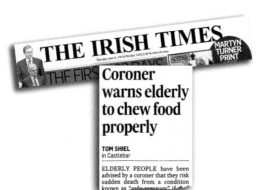

Fig. 4.1

Coroner warns elderly to chew food properly

TOM SHIEL
in Castlebar

ELDERLY PEOPLE have been
advised by a coroner that they risk
sudden death from a condition
known as "café coronary", if a

The Irish Times, *Thursday, June 16, 2011*

Elderly people have been advised by a coroner that they risk sudden death from a condition known as 'café coronary' if they fail to chew food, particularly meat, properly. Dr Eleanor Fitzgerald, acting coroner for north Mayo, gave the warning at an inquest in Ballina into the death of Nora Murphy (81), Currabaggan, Knockmore, Ballina. Ms Murphy was out for Sunday dinner in Hotel Ballina with her husband, Donal, on January 9th when she suddenly slumped in her chair. Efforts by ambulance personnel to revive her failed and she was pronounced dead at the scene. At first it was thought Ms Murphy died from a heart attack or some other medical reason but a postmortem examination later at Mayo General Hospital in Castlebar showed a large intact portion of cooked meat impacted in her larynx. Consultant pathologist Dr Fadel Bennani said victims of what was known as 'café coronary' showed symptoms resembling a heart attack. The condition was well known, Dr Bennani told the hearing, and happened mostly in the elderly and in small children. Returning a verdict of misadventure, the coroner said elderly people especially should be aware of the dangers of eating a large portion of meat. 'This is a warning for the rest of us,' Dr Fitzgerald added. 'We should all be careful to chew food properly.' The medical cause of death was given as asphyxia due to impacted food in the larynx.

This dramatic, frightening and sometimes fatal situation can arise when food is not chewed properly into small pieces before an attempt is made to swallow it. If it is swallowed in one large piece it can become lodged in the throat (larynx), blocking the passage of inhaled air from the mouth or nose so that it cannot reach the lungs. When this happens the person cannot breathe in or out and, if the condition is not relieved very quickly, can literally choke to death. As the sufferers cannot exhale, they are unable to speak and cannot tell others what is happening. Their blood and skin colour will turn a dark blue (a condition known as cyanosis) as a result of their inability to inhale oxygen-containing air. If the blockage is not relieved they will collapse and die, often clasping their chest. This is known as the 'café coronary', because it can happen in restaurants and onlookers often mistakenly think the person is having a heart attack. Sometimes a well-meaning first aider may attempt to press on the person's chest and administer cardiac massage and, worse still, rescue breathing (mouth to mouth resuscitation). By doing this, they can force the impacted food further down the unfortunate victim's airway, a disastrous thing to do in the circumstances.

In 1982 a study of the fatal 'café coronary' was published by Dr Roger Mittleman in *The Journal of the American Medical Association.* It showed a significant association of this condition with denture-wearing and that the risk increased significantly with age, with a peak incidence occurring in those over seventy. In most cases the fatal incidents occurred in a private home or an institution but approximately one third happened in a restaurant and in 85 per cent of those recorded others were present at the time of the incident. Dr R. Wick published a review of victims seen at autopsy in *Journal of Forensic Medicine* in 2006. He recorded that 61 per cent of such victims either had no teeth or had a significant number missing. The most common food culprit in restaurant incidents was meat, when combined with alcohol intake. In the case of institutions, soft foods were often involved, particularly when sedative drugs had been prescribed or in the presence of neurological disease that might affect muscle control.

There have been many calls for a greater awareness of this condition and how to treat it in an emergency. The procedure recommended today is the abdominal thrust, originally known as the 'Heimlich manoeuvre'. Given the fact that so many children are at risk from accidental inhalation of a wide range of objects, including peanuts, small toys, coins and pins, it is a first-aid procedure that is really valuable when correctly applied.

Teeth for life?

A good question to ask is how long is it possible for us to keep our own teeth? The good news is that the trend in Ireland and indeed in all developed countries is a significant increase in the length of time that people keep some or all of their teeth. Several factors have brought about this favourable change, including better dental care and the use of fluorides in toothpaste and in other dental products. Another contributory factor – although a more controversial one – has been the introduction of fluoridation to public water supplies in Ireland.

Adult dental health surveys have produced figures on dental health for the Republic of Ireland. The percentage of the population over the age of fifty-five who have lost all their teeth fell from 72 per cent in 1979 to 45 per cent in 1990. In the latest (2002) *National Survey of Adult Dental Health*, carried out by the Oral Health Services Research Centre, University College Cork, the number had fallen to 41 per cent. (Fig. 4.2) Although this is a positive trend it is clear that the rate

Fig. 4.2

Proportion of older people with no teeth (edentulous) over time

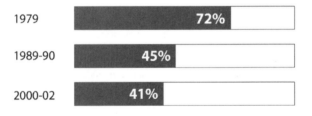

1979	72%
1989-90	45%
2000-02	41%

of improvement is falling off and, as we shall see, the figures may not reveal the true extent of the problems that face an ageing population.

In Ireland the NCAOP (National Council on Ageing and Older People), a statutory body, considered the dental needs of the ageing patient. Entitled 'Evidence-based Options for an Oral Health Policy for Older People', the report was commissioned by the agency in conjunction with the Health Research Board and undertaken by the Oral Health Services Centre, University Dental School and Hospital, Cork. This excellent review evaluates the dental services that will be required, including access to these services for those in residential care, as well as reviewing many of the specific quality-of-life issues and dental problems of the ageing population.

Although many people keep their teeth longer than they might have done in previous decades, this extension will certainly not be able to keep pace with the longer life span of the fastest growing segment of the population. Furthermore, keeping teeth longer may in itself cause a problem if a patient has to wear complete dentures at some stage later in life. The reason for this is that the more elderly the patient the less well able they are to adjust to and manage the bulk of complete dentures, especially as neuromuscular control also diminishes with ageing. The falling off in our ability to learn (neuroplasticity) and in neuromuscular control with ageing are well-recognised phenomena. This is why handwriting deteriorates. The ability to cope with new dentures decreases significantly with age. Dental practitioners and indeed many patients will confirm the difficulties encountered in providing first-time or replacement dentures for elderly patients.

One significant oral health problem many older people will face revolves around something we all take for granted until it is no longer there. This precious substance is saliva.

The difficult problem of dry mouth

Saliva is produced from three sources in the mouth. The first is the large salivary glands, known as the parotid glands, which lie deep in the tissues on each side of the face. The second is the submandibular glands that lie beneath the floor of the mouth. The secretions from these glands pour into the mouth from small ducts or openings in the cheeks and the lining of the mouth beneath the tongue. The third source is the many hundreds of small mucous glands that are embedded in the soft tissues of the mouth; their secretions add to the magic mix that is saliva.

Everyone knows how unpleasant it is to experience a dry mouth: it affects speech, mouth tissues become very sensitive and swallowing food becomes extremely difficult. Mucous secretions provide lubrication that protects the highly sensitive and fragile tissues that line the mouth and prevents food from irritating them. When we chew food it forms a wet, sticky mixture with saliva that allows it to be swallowed easily. The mouth is kept clean and acids that cause decay are neutralised by the twenty-four-hour secretions of saliva that we constantly swallow. Without saliva, food particles are retained in an unpleasant way, especially around the teeth. Saliva also contains many antibodies that help to protect the teeth and gums against disease such as dental decay and gum disease.

Many ill effects result from saliva secretions drying up over an extended period. Many people may have experienced the unpleasant short-term effects of dry mouth (xerostomia) when they have become dehydrated or have overindulged in alcohol. As part of the ageing process, salivary gland function can decline, with changes to the amount, quality and consistency of the saliva being produced. This becomes most noticeable at night and often sufferers will take a glass of water to bed with them to help counteract this unpleasant situation. This natural fall-off in salivary gland function that occurs with age can be made much worse by smoking. It can also be made worse as an unwelcome side effect of taking any one of a wide range of important medicines that may be prescribed for medical conditions associated with ageing. Combinations of such medicines (polypharmacy) are more likely to act in this way. One of the observations emerging from the TILDA studies is the surprisingly large number of medications taken by an ageing population.

A further problem is that dry mouth may be one of the symptoms in many of the diseases that are more common in an ageing population, such as diabetes.

Even in a previously well-cared-for mouth the effects of dry mouth on the teeth can be dramatic, especially if illness or other circumstances now prevent good maintenance. Without the protective influence of saliva, tooth decay may become rampant and attack the root surfaces of teeth. It is not uncommon to see a lifetime of high-quality dentistry, including crowns and bridgework, crumble in the absence of saliva. Artificial saliva products can provide some symptomatic relief from dry mouth problems but at the moment there is no substitute for the real thing.

For those who have lost all their teeth and are wearing dentures the results of a lack of saliva are simply disastrous. Unless dentures develop suction and a good seal against the mouth tissues they will not stay put. In order for this to happen a layer of saliva of the right consistency (viscosity) is required. Dentures will not stay in place without the right amount of saliva and their movement against the dry mouth tissues will irritate them, causing swelling, discomfort and possibly painful ulcers. This may paint a miserable picture but it is not as miserable as the reality. It is not difficult to imagine the challenges that people with such dental problems will have in accessing any kind of varied, healthy and nutritional diet. For older people who live in residential accommodation, without the availability of good dental care, life will be even more miserable.

Unfortunately, it appears that, for many, natural teeth are unlikely to survive long enough to meet the demands of a longer life. For these people, the third age will necessitate a 'third dentition'. The use of dental implants can go a long way to achieving this and, as we will discover, modify many of the otherwise irreversible changes that can cause so much misery and loss of quality of life and even health in older people. Furthermore, old age in itself is no barrier to placing dental implants.

Ageing, dental implants and public health policies

It must be emphasised that this chapter and indeed this book focuses almost entirely on understanding the effects of the loss of all or most of one's teeth. There can be no doubt that implants can play a significant role in improving function and the quality of life, by preventing bone loss and improving self-esteem and aesthetics as we grow older. It must be stressed, however, that oral health problems in those who are getting older are very much wider than the scope of this book and, as with all health problems, public health policies must concentrate on prevention. This includes addressing the negative effects on the mouth tissues of smoking and other lifestyle choices such as diet and alcohol. It is important to identify and adopt effective and affordable strategies to help patients enjoy good oral health, free of disease. The goal is to retain a minimum of twenty healthy teeth, as recommended by WHO.

Clearly, when economic resources for healthcare are very much under pressure, priorities must be established. The particular problem of oral hygiene and oral health in institutionalised elderly patients and in those with special needs is of the greatest importance. In *Journal of the Irish Dental Association*, July 2010, Professor Finbar Allen states: 'a major challenge for the dental profession will be to plan oral healthcare for older adults that is affordable, readily accessible and that positively impacts on the quality of life'. Priorities must be established. These must arise from careful evidence-based research of needs and policies, such as the TILDA project, if they are to provide for this rapidly growing sector in our society. Currently the HSE is undertaking a *National Oral Health Policy Review* that will look at aspects of dental and oral health care in Ireland.

Our own published multi-centre study undertaken in Trinity College Dublin, the Royal College of Surgeons in Ireland and Queen's University Belfast has shown that dentures supported by implants improve the quality of life of patients in comparison to those who are wearing conventional dentures. However, this is not the end of the story as studies have also shown that improving function with good dentures or dentures supported by implants does not necessarily result in a better diet. It would seem that once a semi-liquid diet has established itself as result of loss of function it does not automatically change when chewing function is restored, unless the social conditions and ability to do so are favourable. It is also a fact that many elderly patients do not wish to have implants, as they do not wish to undergo surgery.

When looking at cost-effective ways to help an elderly population by means of dental implants it is important that only interventions that have an evidence base to show they are safe and beneficial over time should be considered. Reducing the cost, minimising the extent of any surgical intervention and simplifying the denture or the teeth that attach to the implants are challenges that are currently being explored.

5

When Appearance Becomes a Matter of Life and Death

*'Luckless that I am!' said Don Quixote, hearing the sad
news his squire gave him; 'I had rather they despoiled me
of an arm, so it were not the sword-arm; for I tell thee,
Sancho, a mouth without teeth is like a mill without
a millstone and a tooth is much more to be prised
than a diamond.'*
Miguel de Cervantes (1547-1616), *Don Quixote*, 1605

In Chapter 3 we looked at the changes in the quantity and quality of the facial bones that occur when natural teeth are lost. Not surprisingly, when such changes happen to these deep supportive structures they also have an impact on the muscles of the face. Facial contours can alter dramatically. It may seem unbelievable but in the 16th century, many young women were burnt at the stake as a result of losing all their teeth prematurely and the facial changes that resulted. How could such a thing happen?

You normally close your jaws by moving your lower jaw towards the upper one. The movement will stop when your teeth meet. At this point the face achieves its normal vertical dimension and in this way a specific distance is maintained between the tip of the nose and the tip of the chin. This dimension is in harmony with and in proportion to the distance between your nose and your eyes. This vertical dimension, along with the support that the lips give to the teeth, provides a pleasing youthful appearance, as can be seen in Fig. 5.1.

However, when no teeth are present, the lower jaw will over-close because there is no longer a natural buffer to prevent the lower jaw moving on towards the upper jaw. The chin will consequently move much closer to the tip of the nose. This has the effect of shortening the lower third of the face, giving an appearance of premature ageing.

With the continuing loss of the underlying jawbone, the overlying tissues and musculature of the face lose support and begin to sag. When there are no teeth, the cheeks sink inward and the lips lose their fullness. Instead of having nice rounded contours with a cupid's bow, the lips come to resemble a featureless horizontal opening. Lines develop between the tip of the nose and corner of the mouth and small vertical lines appear around the lips. The chin also appears to become more prominent. When this happens in a younger person they can end up looking much older than their chronological age, whereas older people who have managed to keep their teeth, or had replacements, can look much younger than their years (Fig. 5.2, Fig. 5.3).

In extreme cases the facial changes following tooth loss can produce the 'witch face' we see every Hallowe'en in masks and posters: collapsed cheeks, long overhanging nose and upward-pointed protruding chin practically meeting the nose. It's what immediately

Fig. 5.1

Licensed from Publitek Inc. dba, Fotosearch 21155, Watertown Road, Waukesha, WI 53186, USA.

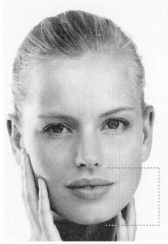

Vertical Dimension

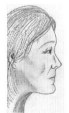 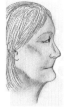 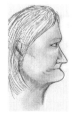 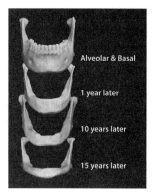

Fig. 5.2

Fig 5.3

© *Professor David Harris: artist Lia Cowan.*

© *Paul Harris.*

comes to mind when the word 'hag' is used.

The witch face is an inevitable long-term consequence of tooth loss that is not rehabilitated. The mouth shrinks inward, creating 'drawstring wrinkles' around the lips. The extra movement and difficulty in eating puts increased work on the muscles of the chin, which tend to get larger as a result. This further emphasises the aged appearance.

These changes were well described by Cervantes in his description of the 'knight of the rueful countenance', who had a permanently sad appearance after he lost his incisors and molar teeth (Fig. 5.4). Don Quixote may have looked sad as a result of his tooth loss but at least his life would not have been endangered by it, as happened to a generation of unfortunate women all over Europe.

When Europe became inflamed by the witch craze in the fifteenth and sixteenth centuries, any particularly noticeable aspect of a woman's appearance made her vulnerable to witch hunters convinced that she was a threat to Christianity. Young women who had lost all their teeth, or perhaps did not develop any in the first place, would develop a 'witch' appearance through no fault of their own. This was considered to be a sure sign of a witch. It was widely believed that such women met at night in covens, cast satanic spells on anyone who crossed them and could fly on their own broomsticks. The very fact

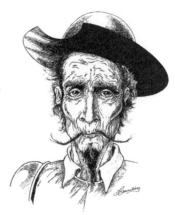

Fig 5.4

© *'Don Quixote's Countenance after Losing his Teeth'. Reproduced with permission of* Journal of Dental Research.

that many older women had cats as pets became an identifier: see, she has a black cat; it's really the devil in feline form.

It didn't help that some of these women had genuine knowledge of the functioning of herbs. They knew how to heal cuts, set bones and ease the pain of childbirth. They were a community resource. Unfortunately, the community used them for evil as well as for good purposes. If you had a fight with a neighbour, a key step in putting him in his place might be a visit to the local 'wise woman' to seek a spell to make his cows go off their feed or his hens stop laying. The wise woman looked the part, with her shrunken old face, even though she might be only in her thirties.

When the witch frenzy began, a version of the Inquisition happened in one community after another. 'Witch finders' authorised by the Church would arrive into the neighbourhood and set up shop. They tended to operate a divide-and-conquer policy, inviting people to save their own skins by informing on others. The easiest potential victims were isolated old widows meddling with cauldrons of herbal preparations. Suddenly, neighbours who had sought out these old women for medical and other help decided that they were witches and denounced them to the witch finders. The next step was an ostensibly fair trial, which was, in reality, anything but fair. The old woman – the woman who had assisted mothers giving birth, shown them how to nurse, the woman who had cleaned wounds and covered them with honey, an effective anti-bacterial – was strapped to a chair which was lowered into the local river. If she floated, then the devil was with her and the case against her was considered proven. She was guilty and was removed from the river and burned at the stake. If, on the other hand she drowned, she was deemed to have been innocent.

We should not underestimate the number of women who became victims of mass hysteria at this time. *The European Witch-Craze of the Sixteenth and Seventeenth Centuries* (1969), the seminal account by Hugh Trevor-Roper (1914-2003) of this grim period in history, established that, in many countries, communities were left with only a tiny minority of women because of the contamination of panic. To try to save themselves, women informed on other women who had never done anything wrong and hundreds of thousands of them (together with some men) were tortured and burned. People today sometimes say that men bond more easily with one another than do women and trust one another more; it has been suggested that this can be traced back to a time when to be a woman who had knowledge and friends was to be endangered and to be a woman who had lost her teeth was to be acutely endangered.

Queen Elizabeth I (1533-1603) was so concerned when she lost her teeth, with the result that her cheeks became hollow and her lips wrinkled, that she took to stuffing her face with rolls of cloth when making public appearances. This must have greatly interfered with her diction. But remember, the last twenty years of this woman's life coincided with the onset of the European witch craze. She had survived chaotic times and many threats since her birth and lived in a period when poor diction mattered a lot less than looking like a witch.

For those affluent enough to be able to afford it, the European diet grew less healthy for teeth and gums. In the 18th century refined carbohydrates in the form of white bread became more common and also the use of sugar as a sweetener. Many who could afford it developed a 'sweet tooth', a preference for sugary foods. This meant a great deal more tooth decay and, as a result, a demand for many more professional dentists. Barber surgeons and travelling tooth extractors originally carried out dentistry, travelling from town to town offering 'painless extractions'. The extractions often took place in public squares and the practitioners were accompanied by a small troop of musicians who played loudly to drown out the cries of their 'patients'. The extractions must have been extremely painful and people needed to be desperate to suffer them in order to put an end to the pain of the decayed teeth.

Around the middle of the 18th century, the practice of dentistry began to develop as a recognised profession in Europe and North America, having originated in France. Human and animal teeth were in great demand and attached to ingenious devices to replace missing teeth. Perhaps the most famous replacement teeth were the set of dentures made for the first American president, George Washington (1732-99), which were hand-carved from ivory with a combination of human and animal teeth. They had springs attached, which pushed the dentures apart in an attempt to stop them from falling out. Fig. 5.5 illustrates the type of denture worn by George Washington and Fig. 5.6 his appearance.

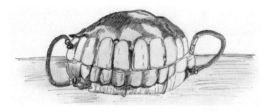

Fig 5.5

© Professor David Harris: artist Lia Cowan.

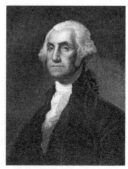

Fig 5.6

Portrait of President George Washington reproduced under licence from iStockphoto LP. Suite 200, 1240 20th Ave SE, Calgary, Alberta, T2G 1M8, Canada.

The problem with teeth carved from ivory or animal bone was that they were subject to degradation from the acid and bacteria produced in the mouth. They often became foul smelling, as did the untreated gum disease of people who still had their own teeth. It seems that one of the functions of a fan in times past was to mask the terrible odour that resulted from decayed teeth and gum infections.

The availability of dentists and the ever-growing demand for teeth replacements opened up a business opportunity for their supply. It was considered that healthy human teeth were the most suitable for use as replacements as they would last longer and look much better than those made from animal tissue. Such teeth were most likely to be found in young, healthy adults. The Napoleonic Wars in Europe (1803-15) and the Civil War in America (1861-5) provided the necessary material for this gruesome trade.

Napoleon Bonaparte (1769-1821) should figure in any history of dental health. His own toothbrush is on display in the Royal College of Physicians' building in Kildare Street in Dublin. Pathetic and ineffective as it looks, the very fact that he owned a toothbrush indicated a concern for his teeth – a concern that matched his interest, at least in the early days, for the health of his army. 'An army marches on its stomach,' was one of his famous statements. He understood that well-nourished men fought well. The Duke of Wellington (1769-1852) had markedly less respect for the fighting force he brought to Waterloo. 'I have an infamous army,' he remarked. This infamous army nevertheless beat Napoleon into submission in 1815, leaving fifty thousand dead on the field of battle.

A couple of months later, an English barrister named Henry Crabb Robinson toured the flat, treeless plain of Waterloo, where the disintegrating bodies of the dead were being ground up for fertiliser. This was after they had been looted of their swords and boots – and dispossessed of their teeth.

If you think about it, young soldiers needed good teeth so they could chew their food. Hence the teeth obtained from those fallen in the battlefield were considered to be the best obtainable. In the aftermath of battle there were always those who plundered the fallen and they added teeth to their list of plundered items such as jewellery. An excellent article by Stephanie Pain entitled 'The Great Tooth Robbery' in *New Scientist* magazine of 16 June 2001 sums up the situation perfectly:

Taking teeth from the dead to replace those lost by the living was nothing new. But this time the scale was different. The flood of teeth on to the market was so huge that dentures made from second-hand teeth acquired a new name: 'Waterloo teeth'. Far from putting clients off, this was a positive selling point. Better to have teeth from a relatively fit and healthy young man killed by a cannonball or sabre than incisors plucked from the jaws of a disease-ridden corpse decaying in a grave or from a hanged man left dangling too long on the gibbet.

Some months after visiting the battlefield, Henry Crabb Robinson himself became the recipient of a 'Waterloo tooth'. His dentist seems to have been good at marketing. 'He assured me it came from Waterloo,' the barrister confided to his diary, 'and promised me it should outlast twelve artificial teeth.'

Early dental transplants

Because losing their teeth posed a real and present danger of death to humans living millennia ago, they imagined the possibility of setting something into the gums that would allow them to eat again and did their best to create primitive dental implants. The Mayans in Mexico and Central America were known to have carried out dental implantations: a 1300-year-old jawbone was found in Honduras, which had implants of tooth-shaped shells. Examination of the skulls of Egyptian mummies has revealed gold wires inserted in the sockets of missing teeth.

In Europe the earliest recorded dental implant was discovered in the remains of a Roman soldier in a Gallo-Roman necropolis at Chatambre (Essone, France). An upper-right second premolar tooth made of wrought iron had been perfectly fitted into the jawbone.

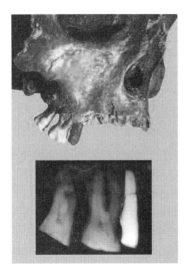

Fig. 5.7

Reprinted with permission of Nature Publishing Group and Dr Eric Cruzby. (Nature, Vol. 391, January 1st 1998, p.29: 'False Teeth of the Roman World'.)

These remains, shown in Fig. 5.7, were dated to the first or second century AD.

The history of creating permanent replacement teeth by transplantation is one of exploitation and failure. The exploitation was of impoverished young people. Nineteenth-century cartoons showed skinny boys and girls – domestic servants and stable boys – waiting to have their perfectly healthy teeth wrested from their mouths by surgeons who wished to replace the diseased teeth they had just removed from rich old people. The idea was that the young person's tooth would be transplanted straight into the hole left by the extraction in the older person's gums and bone, where it might take root. The young person was glad of the money. The older person had a brand new tooth.

The short-term success of such transplants was poor. Quite apart from the fact that, as operating conditions were appallingly unsterile, infections were a constant hazard, there would have been frequent rejection of the strange new arrival in a mouth full of diseased teeth. This didn't stop the surgeons of the time claiming phenomenal success, even though they tended to run out of young people willing, even for a few shillings, to sacrifice their teeth and undergo the horror of extraction without any anaesthetic. There was talk of taking teeth from animals instead and 'resurrectionists', who invaded graveyards to disinter the recently deceased, were sometimes motivated by the possibility of selling the cadavers' teeth to dental surgeons.

The notoriety of men like Burke and Hare put an end to the purchase by surgeons of dead bodies or parts thereof. Burke and Hare, who operated in Edinburgh in the late 1820s, went beyond digging up dead bodies, deciding that killing people was a simpler way of supplying fresh corpses for anatomical study. They were caught and convicted. This meant that dental transplants based on teeth from cadavers ceased to be an option. This trade really came to an end in the 1840s, with the invention and availability of totally artificial porcelain teeth.

The tipping point

Up to this point, Crabb Robinson's dentist had been correct: when replacement teeth were fashioned of copper, pearls, walrus teeth, elephant ivory, cattle bones or wood, they tended to be neither comfortable nor durable. Even when they were expensive works of art, like the set crafted for Lord Hervey (1757-96), son of the 'Earl Bishop' of Derry – Italian craft workers made his false teeth out of agate – history does not record how well they worked for him.

It was not until the mid-19th century that the first modern artificial teeth made their appearance thanks to the discovery of vulcanised rubber. Dentures made of this material could be processed and individually moulded to fit the contours of a patient's mouth. This technique provided a firm base that could adhere to gum tissues or the palate and to which the replacement teeth could be attached.

The 'tipping point' (a term coined by Malcolm Gladwell in his book of that name, published in 2000) for the more widespread acceptability of extractions and dentures occurred with the development of anaesthesia by two dentists named Horace Wells (1815-48) and William Morton (1819-68). As denture-making improved, dentists found themselves with something to sell that nobody wanted to buy because of the pain of the intervening step – the extraction of teeth. Horace Wells and William Morton were particularly frustrated. They had developed improved false teeth and invented a dental solder but not even their 'money back if not satisfied' guarantee could persuade people already missing many of their teeth to undergo the agony of having the remainder removed. The two started to search for something – anything – that would prevent that agony and allow them to increase sales of false teeth.

They got an unexpected Christmas present when, in December 1844, Wells went to a lecture about nitrous oxide or 'laughing gas'. As part of the lecture, a man from the audience agreed to have the gas administered to him. Because he was then intoxicated, he fell off the stage and hurt himself quite badly but Wells noted that he did not appear to be in pain as might be expected. On the contrary, the accident victim seemed to find the incident riotously funny and to experience no discomfort at all.

A light went on in the head of Horace Wells. This gas might have potential in dentistry. At the end of the lecture, he approached the lecturer and asked him to bring the gas to his office the following day, saying that he would submit himself to an experiment. The lecturer, Gardner Quincy Colton (1814-96), duly arrived and anaesthetised Wells and a dental student took out one of his teeth. When Horace Wells came back to consciousness, he was thrilled to realise that he had experienced painless dentistry. He had no recollection at all of having the tooth removed. Even more positively, he had no memory of the pain involved. As soon as Christmas was over, Horace Wells went to work with a will. In the first fortnight of the new year, 1845, he operated, using nitrous oxide, on more than a dozen patients.

It wasn't all plain sailing. The two dentists, triumphant because of their happy patients, decided to demonstrate the anaesthetic gas to medical colleagues at a public event. Unfortunately for them, the patient moaned and thrashed around mid-operation. When he regained consciousness, the cause of the moaning remained a mystery, because he could not remember experiencing any pain. But the damage was done. The medical authorities said that the new 'painless dentistry' had not proven itself to meet the criteria for perfect analgesia (inability to feel pain stimuli). Morton became impoverished. Wells became depressed and began to sniff addictive preparations and behave oddly. He had to be admitted into an asylum for the insane and eventually he committed suicide.

What he and Morton had failed to realise was that nitrous oxide is a very weak anaesthetic, albeit a very safe one. It is unpredictable in its effects. Many patients did not become fully anaesthetised and instead became excited and uncontrollable when it was administered to them. Although they might not retain any memory of the event, they could not be operated on. To this day nitrous oxide is used as a basis for anaesthesia because of its safety and the speed with which it is eliminated from the body. However, it is always deployed in combination with modern anaesthetic agents that ensure that the patient remains unconscious throughout the procedure.

Although the value of Wells's contribution was eventually seen and he was recognised as the discoverer of modern anaesthesia, this recognition was posthumous. His former colleague, dismayed by the setback with nitrous oxide, kept searching for a form of analgesia that would work for dental patients. Most dentists could administer nothing better than laudanum or alcohol, both of which had dangerous side effects. Morton developed an inhaler for ether, which allowed a successful operation on a patient suffering from cancer of the tongue, but then ran into problems because he wouldn't admit the drug used was ether. If he had, anyone could have used it and he would not have earned a single cent from his research. Instead, he disguised it by using a brand name.

This didn't work, because in the US at the time the rules of the medical profession precluded the use of 'secret remedies', so other dentists and doctors could not try out Morton's 'Letheon Gas'. Morton died in the middle of a series of court cases he was taking against people who had, he believed, stolen a proprietary medicine he had developed.

With the availability of well-fitting vulcanite dentures and the development first of general anaesthesia and subsequently of local anaesthesia, the scene was now set for extracting hopeless, decayed and painful teeth and replacing them with dentures.

As we will see, these advances would turn out to be a two-edged sword. They provided undoubted benefits, notably painless extraction of teeth, but they left grave problems in their wake. Those problems were unfortunately complicated by another ostensible gain for humanity. People began to live longer. The scene was set for a subtle tragedy: large numbers of older people handicapped for the later years of their long life by being dental amputees.

6

Non-Implant Methods
of Replacing Missing Teeth

When we lose any of our teeth various options are open to us. One of these is to do nothing, leave well enough alone and accept the loss. It might be surprising to hear a dentist say this but if chewing ability is still satisfactory and the loss does not affect the outlook for any remaining teeth it can be a perfectly reasonable choice. However, for many people this choice can lead to problems in the longer term that may result in further loss of teeth, function and, of course, appearance. This can be true even if only one tooth is lost. The reason for this is that teeth are not fixed into the jawbone. Far from it! They can and do move and shift their position within the mouth – even in adults.

Tooth movement and tooth loss

Teeth lie within jawbone tooth sockets but are separated from the bone by tiny fibres that connect the root of the tooth to the bone. These fibres form a cradle around the root and are known as the periodontal ligament. One of the functions of this ligament is to act as a 'shock absorber' and allow teeth to make very small movements during chewing. When prolonged small pressures are applied to a tooth this ligament will allow a tooth to move through the bone in a direction that will relieve this pressure. The ligament can do this as it contains unique cells that will dissolve bone in the direction that the tooth moves in and, at the same time, cause new bone to form on the opposite side (Fig. 6.1). When the right pressure is applied a tooth can be made to move in any direction.

This is exactly how braces (orthodontic bands) can produce move-

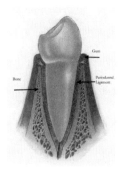
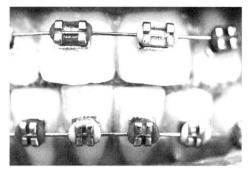

Fig. 6.1 Fig. 6.2

ment of teeth by directing controlled pressure to the teeth. Orthodontic bands and devices allow teeth to be straightened and aligned,
with a view to producing better function and appearance (Fig. 6.2).

Of course teeth have pressure applied to them all the time. They
will normally take up a position that provides a balance between the
pressure of the lips and cheeks on one side and the tongue on the other.
This position will be stabilised and limited by the presence of adjacent
teeth. Another important stabilising factor comes into play when
upper and lower teeth meet, usually during swallowing. Surprisingly,
teeth rarely meet during chewing. When a tooth is lost these stabilising
influences – the adjacent teeth and the opposing tooth in the opposite
jaw – may be lost. The result is that the teeth on either side of the gap
can begin to tilt into the space left and the tooth in the opposite jaw
may start to erupt further into this space. It may surprise some people
that teeth continue to erupt, even in adults.

This effect may remain confined to the immediate area where the
tooth loss has occurred or, over time, can result in other teeth starting
to drift as they seek to find a new balance. The more teeth that are lost
the more severe the effects are likely to be. Sometimes the first thing a
patient will notice is loss of appearance of front teeth that can begin
to overlap, become more prominent or rotated. Slight movements can
cause small spaces to open up and result in trapping of food between
teeth that can cause decay, bad odour and gum disease. A further
unpleasant outcome may result from the upper and lower teeth no

longer meeting in a harmonious way: this can trigger changes in the joint at the point where the lower jaw meets the skull just in front of the ear, the temporomandibular joint (TMJ). Such changes can lead to a clicking or grating noise when the jaws are opened and closed and may be associated with severe headaches and pain in the facial region.

When it is safe not to replace missing teeth?

There are, however situations when the effects of tooth loss are not serious. Sometimes, when a single tooth is lost, the opposing tooth and the adjacent teeth can maintain their position providing that there is some remaining contact with an opposing tooth. When this happens and the patient is not complaining about any loss of function or appearance, matters can be left alone.

It is also true that we do not need a full set of teeth to function well with our modern cooked (pre-digested) diet. Our ancestors may have required teeth and large jaws for grinding hard, rough and uncooked foods but this is not the case nowadays.

A full set of teeth can be considered to be twenty-eight. It is possible to lose eight of these without incurring any drifting or real, measurable loss of function but you cannot lose just any eight teeth. If all the upper and lower molars are missing but the others are intact, the outcome can be a reduced dental arch that is stable and functions well. However, the loss of certain teeth will be more deleterious than others. For example the large canine teeth, so beloved of vampire stories, are particularly important. These cause the back teeth to come apart when the lower jaw moves from side to side and prevent damage from grinding which can wear the enamel down.

Fig. 6.3 and Fig. 6.4 show a patient who is missing a single lower molar. However, the adjacent teeth and the opposing upper teeth are maintaining good contact. In this situation the teeth are stable and there is no need to consider a replacement unless the patient notices a loss of function or feels their appearance is adversely affected – both of which are unlikely in this case.

Apart from these types of exceptions, failure to replace missing

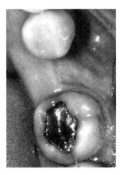
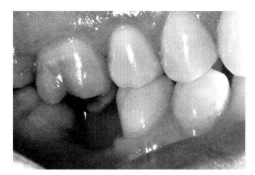

Fig. 6.3   Fig. 6.4

teeth is often the first step on a road that, over time, can lead to the eventual loss of all teeth. This is especially so if the loss arises as a result of gum disease that has not been diagnosed or successfully treated. It is interesting to note that gum disease can affect more than teeth. There is increasing evidence that the type of inflammation associated with gum and periodontal disease is also associated with hardening of the arteries, coronary artery disease and Type 2 diabetes, as well as some indications that it may be a possible contributory factor to rheumatoid arthritis.

Conventional treatment options available when a few teeth have been lost

Patients have two choices available to them: either do nothing and accept the situation as it is or consider replacement teeth. Replacement teeth can be provided in three different ways:

1. as removable dentures
2. as bridgework supported by adjacent teeth
3. as bridgework or crowns supported by dental implants

Dentures

Let us first consider dentures. Patients and dentists alike generally view these as the least desirable long-term option. Although a small denture replacing one or two teeth for cosmetic purposes may do the job, there are drawbacks. A denture consists of artificial teeth that are attached to an acrylic (plastic) or metal plate. Because of this they are more bulky than the teeth they replace. Very many people, especially teenagers and young adults, find that adapting to the bulk of the denture is challenging and having to remove a denture on a daily basis for cleaning is distressing. It is a constant reminder to them that they are not 'complete' and are different from other people.

The success of a denture very much depends on the type of denture that is used. Dentures can range from a simple piece of plastic (acrylic) that lies against the roof of the mouth and gums (Fig. 6.5), to a metal casting with clasps that gain support from other teeth or crowns (Fig. 6.6). A well-made denture can help prevent drifting and over-eruption of teeth but will need replacing at regular intervals. At worst, a simple plastic denture with no tooth support, such as is often described by dentists as a 'gum stripper', should be considered only as a temporary solution. Larger dentures can require a long period to be accustomed to with regard to speech and anyone with a low gag reflex threshold can find them particularly difficult to manage.

In all cases it is vitally important that the gum around the teeth that is covered by a denture is regularly cleaned and well maintained if gum disease is to be avoided. The reason that dentures pose such a problem for the health of the gum tissues may not be immediately obvious. There is a thin band of gum around teeth that needs to be stimulated with brushing or floss or other cleaning aid, if it is to remain healthy. This can be seen as the band of lighter pink colour that lies next to

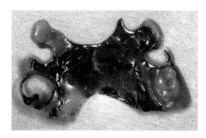

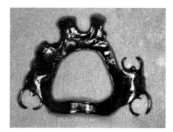

Fig. 6.5   Fig. 6.6

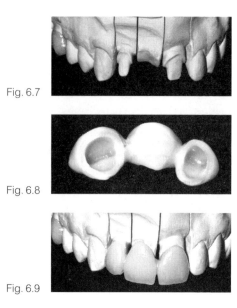

Fig. 6.7

Fig. 6.8

Fig. 6.9

the crowns of healthy teeth. The colour comes from a substance called keratin that thickens and hardens the gums. It is the same process that causes the skin in the hands to thicken in response to working with them. Everyone is familiar with what happens when a first aid plaster is placed on a cut in a finger. Some days later, when the plaster is removed the skin underneath looks white, soggy and soft. The same process occurs under a denture that covers gum and that is why it is so necessary to stimulate the tissues as part of a daily cleaning regime – mouthwashes and toothpaste alone will not do the job. Failure to do so will result in soft, bleeding gums, which are an early sign of deeper gum disease developing.

Bridgework

The second alternative is to consider bridgework. In a bridge the missing tooth (or teeth) is attached to the teeth in front of and behind the gap. This bridgework incorporates crowns that are then fixed to the supporting teeth by dental cement (Fig. 6.7, Fig. 6.8 and Fig. 6.9). In conventional bridgework the supporting teeth have to be prepared, which means that tooth enamel is removed.

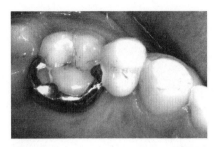

Fig. 6.10

Sometimes adhesive bridgework is used. This follows the same principle as conventional bridgework except that the supporting teeth do not need to be crowned. There is minimal preparation of the tooth enamel, which is etched with an acid to produce a surface similar in appearance to frosted glass. The bridge is then bonded to the etched surface, using specially developed bonding materials. This type of bridge relies on the adhesive properties of the bond to stay in place (Fig. 6.10).

From a patient's point of view a bridge has the advantage that, unlike a denture, it does not have to be removed for cleaning on a daily basis. It is far less bulky than a denture and, as a result, it is usually easier to get used to and causes less interference with speech. Because it does not cover the gum tissues it causes less harm. However, a well-designed bridge must leave adequate space for cleaning and oral hygiene. It is distressing to see patients with poorly designed and contoured bridgework and crowns that have no provision for cleaning and hygiene between the teeth. In such a situation, the treatment provided does not prolong the life of the teeth but encourages the development of disease that will lead to their premature loss. This is known as 'iatrogenic' disease, as it is the treatment itself that has caused the problem. It is sometimes seen when extensive cosmetic treatment with veneers and crowns has been poorly carried out and the patient does not become aware of the problem until much later.

These are some of the disadvantages of bridgework:

• There must be enough teeth on either side of the gap to support the bridge.

- Conventional bridgework is destructive to the supporting teeth, especially if they have never previously been filled.
- A small proportion of teeth used to support the bridgework may go on to develop an abscess and require a root filling to be carried out, something that can further weaken the tooth.
- Patients whose teeth have a high decay rate, or who fail to maintain excellent oral hygiene, are likely to develop decay or gum disease around and under the supporting teeth.

Bridgework is a highly sensitive technique that requires excellent technical support from a laboratory. Ten to fifteen years is the accepted life span for a well-made bridge that is carefully maintained. If decay affects the supporting teeth it may not be possible to remake the bridge. When many teeth have to be replaced, bridgework can become complicated and difficult and have a shorter life span. Additionally, bone loss and gum shrinkage can occur underneath the bridge in the area where teeth are missing.

Adhesive bridgework is less destructive but once again it is very technique-sensitive and it is unsuitable for replacing a large number of teeth. Its main disadvantage is that the bonding can fail, causing the bridge to fall out, usually without warning. If the bridge is replacing teeth towards the front of the mouth, this can be very embarrassing. It is, however, a very valuable option and when well carried out it can be the treatment of choice – especially in younger patients.

As in all areas of restorative dentistry, a thorough examination of the gum tissue and all the remaining teeth is required. The patient's commitment to maintaining good oral hygiene is an absolute pre-requisite in establishing whether or not they will benefit from treatment.

Options when all or most teeth have been lost

For patients who have lost all or a great many of their teeth and who are not candidates for bridgework, the replacement options available become significantly fewer and must involve the use of a denture.

Having a few remaining teeth can be useful in improving the results that can be obtained with a well-constructed denture. Additionally, the presence of some teeth will continue to stimulate the jawbone and prevent or reduce the continuous bone loss that is so destructive. Over the years, observant dental practitioners have recognised the value of preserving a few remaining roots of teeth even when the crowns have been lost as a result of decay. A denture can be made that attaches to these roots or simply rests on them and that can function for a further five to ten years without any bone loss occurring. Such a denture is known as an overdenture.

When all teeth have been lost, the only option is a complete denture (Fig. 6.11). From a functional point of view, well-made dentures can provide excellent results for many patients in the medium term but some will never be able to adapt to them or use them successfully, especially when there is insufficient bone support. The lower denture causes most problems, as there is so little space between the lips and the tongue for the denture to rest on. It is not uncommon to hear patients report that they wear their lower dentures only on social occasions and leave them out whenever they can. Those with a complete upper denture usually cope better, as the upper denture can gain substantial support from the palate. Even with considerable bone loss, many people can continue to function with an upper denture. However very advanced bone loss gives an upper denture an impossible problem to surmount, even with the best-made denture in the world and the use of denture adhesives.

Fig. 6.11

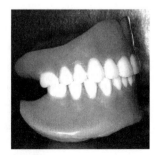

Mouth cancer

There are also important issues with regard to the detrimental effects of dentures that are not well maintained, become ill fitting and are not replaced at suitable intervals. This is especially the case for older people. In western countries, including Ireland, cancer of the mouth is on the increase, accounting for about 5 per cent of all malignant tumours. It is most common in those aged over fifty-five. Many cancers will make their appearance in what appear to be healthy tissues but most will arise from tissues that show early signs of developing malignant cancer. These are known as 'premalignant' lesions and commonly take the form of a white patch or a red area. If these are discovered early and monitored or treated, full-blown cancer can be prevented and the lesions treated without the extensive surgery and adjunctive treatment necessary for advanced cases. This topic lies outside the remit of this book but the role of ill-fitting dentures in the development of cancer of the mouth needs to be highlighted.

Any source of chronic irritation in the mouth has the potential to generate pre-malignant changes. Dentures that may be well fitting initially will not change their shape when bone and gum begin to shrink and will begin to dig into the soft tissues of the mouth. This may result in ulcers forming on the gums or a localised tissue swelling may form which may subsequently become ulcerated. Over time, a small number of these can develop into premalignant lesions, especially when combined with smoking and high alcohol intake. Although these ulcers may be painful, often they are not so painful and patients ignore them. When dentures are the cause they need to be trimmed back so they no longer impinge on the tissues. The area should be carefully monitored and, if necessary, a biopsy taken to identify whether there is anything to worry about. This involves a small amount of tissue being removed and examined with special dyes under a microscope. Wearers of complete dentures need to attend for dental check-ups and at varying intervals have the dentures relined so they fit well to the changing contours in the mouth – or if necessary have a new set made.

Mouth Cancer Awareness Day

Each year some three hundred cases of oral cancer are diagnosed in Ireland. Sadly, a number of these turn out to be quite advanced when diagnosed and can require extensive and debilitating treatment. The advantages of early diagnosis at the premalignant stage are obvious and hugely beneficial. The Irish Dental Association promotes a Mouth Cancer Awareness Day each year, when dentists throughout the country will provide oral cancer screening free of charge to anyone – even if they are not patients of the practice. This excellent initiative by the Irish Dental Association has benefitted many patients. Whereas the vast majority of those examined are found to have no problems a referral process is in place in the Dental Schools in Dublin and Cork and the National Maxillofacial Unit in St James's Hospital in Dublin where any suspicious findings can be thoroughly investigated.

Inflammation and Infections

Inflammation and infections can occur in the tissues on which dentures rest: this is commonly referred to as 'denture sore mouth'. The medical term is 'denture induced stomatitis'. It is more common in older people. The tissues appear red and inflamed, with the inflammation usually confined to the area of the mouth covered by the denture. Plastic dentures are porous and it is relatively easy for bacteria and fungi to take up residence in them. Many different organisms may be involved but the most commonly associated with denture-induced stomatitis is the fungus *candida albicans*, popularly known as thrush. In severe cases yeast colonies can appear in the mouth as whitish plaques adherent to the mucosa. It is more common in those suffering from dry mouth. It can also spread to the corners of the mouth and lips, where it will appear as a reddish lesion visible from the outside and is known as angular cheilitis. Treatment of this condition usually involves soaking the dentures at night in an antifungal solution and the prescription of a suitable antifungal medication. This condition is sometimes associated with iron-deficiency anaemia as well as deficiencies in vitamins such as folic acid and B complex.

Clearly, dentures are less than ideal replacements for missing teeth, especially complete dentures. Dental implants offer an alternative approach. They prevent many of the problems outlined and hold out the possibility of long-term comfort and function as well as the preservation of the jawbone. They are the nearest we can get to having a third set of teeth.

7

Per-Ingvar Brånemark
and the Modern Dental Implant

The man whose name is synonymous, world-wide, with the development of modern dental implants, made his big breakthrough because of a fortuitous observation, hated the phrase 'implant' and was never a dental surgeon. He did, however, change the history of dental surgery worldwide and transform the quality of lives – and in some cases the longevity – of people who had lost all their teeth. He managed to make a dream that goes back to ancient times a reality.

The idea of the dental implant has been around for more than two thousand years and some of the more bizarre ways in which the idea was put into practice are described in Chapter 5. Such early experiments never led to a continuum of successful implants and, unfortunately, the pattern of one-off success followed by abandonment of the idea continued into modern times.

The 20th century saw more serious attempts to design and use 'modern' dental implants. The period 1950-70 was particularly notable for the increasing number of innovators attempting to produce viable dental implants that might provide long-term function. Many ingenious mechanical designs of different shapes, sizes and materials were introduced into clinical dentistry and surgically placed within patients' jawbones. Societies were formed to promote the new 'science' of implantology and different groups enthusiastically promoted particular types of implants. Sadly, in spite of the good intentions of all concerned, the reality was that most of these implants had little or no research to support their use and so amounted to nothing more than human experimentation. With so many dental amputees desperate for help there was certainly no shortage of patients willing to undergo these procedures. The results were disastrous. It became clear that Mother Nature would not collaborate with mechanical ingenuity that does not take into account the biological necessities that are essential for success.

Although some of these implants appeared to work well for a short period, they were all doomed to failure, as the body's own immune system eventually rejected them as a foreign body. During the rejection process the bone and soft tissues surrounding the implant became inflamed. Scar tissue formed around the implant in an attempt to isolate the 'intruder' from the surrounding healthy mouth tissues. Eventually, the implant would become exfoliated, loosen and fall out. Sometimes this process was complicated by a localised but serious infection, which caused loss of jawbone itself. It also resulted in scarring of the soft tissues, leaving the mouth tissues in a dreadful, mutilated state. Like many patients who undergo untested, experimental surgery, 'modern' implant patients in the early days often suffered greatly. At best they ended up back where they started or, more often than not, in a significantly worse condition than before the surgery.

This rejection process results from our bodies built-in immune response. Although this response was disastrous for early implant patients, is absolutely essential for life. It enables our bodies to recognise, neutralise and overcome any invasion by foreign substances such as bacteria and viruses, or other harmful challenges. Without it we simply could not survive.

Because of the dreadful medium and long-term results of these early attempts, the vast majority of the dental profession became convinced that dental implants were a crazy idea. They believed that it would never prove possible to place metal or other material in bone, as it would always be regarded as a foreign tissue and eventually rejected by the body. This was all to change with the man who researched and eventually developed osseointegrated implants.

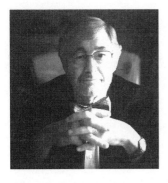

Fig. 7.1

Reproduced by kind permission of Professor P.-I. Brånemark.

Professor Brånemark

The story of modern dental implants that can produce predictable long-term results arose from the meticulous research, ingenuity and dedication of one-man, Professor Per-Ingvar Brånemark (1929-2014) (Fig. 7.1). The following is a short account of his remarkable story.

Brånemark was an anatomical biologist and orthopaedic surgeon, who carried out research in the University of Lund in southern Sweden in the 1950s, examining how various body tissues and especially bone reacted to and recovered from surgical trauma. Brånemark was curious to understand the cellular changes that went on between injured bone itself and the surrounding healthy bone – especially the bone marrow – during healing. In order to observe this process directly, he developed special optical inspection chambers that could be surgically inserted into the bones of animals – in this case, rabbits were used – and connected them to specially designed microscopes. These devices allowed him to directly observe and record bloodflow and any cellular changes that occurred in living tissues as healing progressed. He first choice was to make these chambers from a material called tantalum but this changed to titanium when tantalum proved too difficult to source.

Titanium

Titanium is a hard, silvery-grey metallic element, first discovered in Cornwall in 1791 by a clergyman, the Reverend William Gregor. Initially known as 'menaccanite' after the local Cornish parish of

Menaccan, it was eventually called 'titanium' after the Titans in Greek mythology. Titanium is widely found in countries such as Australia, Russia and Norway, as well as in meteorites, and is present on the moon and the sun. It is as strong as steel but about 45 per cent lighter and twice as strong as aluminium alloys. Metallurgists discovered very early on that titanium is highly resistant to corrosion, especially corrosion arising from being immersed in seawater. These properties, along with its very high melting point, are especially valuable in the marine and aerospace industries. Its resistance to corrosion also attracted the attention of medical researchers who were interested in a metallic substance that might not react when inserted into body tissues – which are themselves corrosive – and might prove to be more biocompatible than other metals.

A former watchmaker, a member of Brånemark's team, worked out ways to create the tiny optical chambers the professor needed to insert into the delicate bones of the rabbits he wanted to study. Because the titanium devices were both difficult and expensive to produce, only a small number were made, with the idea that they would be retrieved and reused many times. The results of the research proved very valuable and interesting, although not quite as interesting as what happened when Brånemark tried to remove these optical chambers: he found he had enormous difficulty separating them from the bone. The bone appeared to have developed a tenacious connection and had grown over and into the surface of the titanium. This was an extraordinary outcome, given the well-known capacity of animal bodies to do exactly the opposite and reject any foreign material introduced into them.

Brånemark was curious about this finding and decided to take a closer look. When he examined the specimens under very high-powered electron microscopy, he observed that not only did the bone cells appear to have a tenacious connection with the surface of the titanium but that the normal inflammatory and rejection process between living bone and the implanted material seemed to have been bypassed. He named this process 'osseointegration' ('osseous' means containing or relating to bone). The Swedish professor realised that this odd, chance finding of a metal that would happily marry with bone might have some potential for medical use. A little like Alexander Fleming, who discovered penicillin in the course of researching something else (when contaminated Petri dishes grew a mould that attacked bacteria), Professor Brånemark realised that, although it had not been the original objective of his research, osseointegration might be of great importance.

He was certainly on to something. Brånemark had identified a material that did not appear to cause adverse reactions in soft tissues and which bone positively welcomed as part of itself. He also realised that this phenomenon had never previously been described. The possibilities were enormous. He decided to extend his research to find out how this bonding could best be achieved in human tissues.

One of Brånemark's great strengths is his capacity to collaborate with others, whether in his own country or in other parts of the world. He soon assembled a team made up of clinicians and researchers who were as curious as he was about a material that could interact with tissues in this way.

It took endless research to discover how titanium should be processed in order to carry out this great subterfuge of getting bone to accept a foreign body. Much of this research was conducted humanely on animals. Brånemark reasoned that it might have a major positive role to play in surgical reconstructions, for example, in the aftermath of motorcycle injuries. He had always believed that surgical procedures and interventions should be carried out as gently as possible, with the minimum of damage or disturbance to the living healthy tissues. He suspected that this, in turn, would result in more rapid and complete healing. In his animal studies he showed that, if gentle surgical techniques were used, bone would predictably integrate (join) with the surface of pure titanium. In order to achieve this it was also necessary to ensure that the titanium itself did not become contaminated and that a healing period of several months should be allowed during which no pressure was applied to the implant. He went on to show that following this healing period the intimate bonding with bone could be maintained and stand up to any functional loads placed on it.

To apply these findings to humans meant taking his experiments to the clinical stage by placing them into the bone of the human skeleton. As it turned out, his experimental work did not start with the larger bones of the body but within the bones of the jaws of people who had lost all their teeth. He was assured of a constant supply of volunteer patients who needed help with dental reconstruction as a result of tooth loss or trauma.

Nor was this the only advantage of placing oral implants. 'From the scientific point of view, the oral cavity is the perfect location for controlled clinical trials,' Brånemark pointed out. 'It's the only area of the body where exploratory procedures are unnecessary. Ask your patient to open his or her mouth and you can inspect the reconstruction region without any difficulty at all. You can go back and see the consequences of your actions.'

The first patient to benefit from dental implants was a man who had a major facial deformity. 'I couldn't even chew a slice of bread,' the patient said. 'The few teeth I had were more or less randomly distributed throughout my head. My jawbone was not very strong either.'

This unfortunate man, named Gösta Larsson, had, by his mid-thirties, learned to cope with his disability. He could neither speak nor eat normally and was resigned to it – until the day his doctor talked to him about becoming a human guinea pig in research designed to explore osseointegration. He indicated that he was willing and went to meet Professor Brånemark. The two men developed a high level of mutual trust and the procedure went ahead. Four titanium implants were fitted into his weak jawbone and, in due course, a bridge of teeth affixed to them.

The change was miraculous. He could talk. He could eat. His appearance radically improved. Nobody knew how long the implanted teeth would survive but as time passed, it became clear that they could become permanent fixtures – so permanent they even survived a car crash. Twenty-five years after he received dental implants, Larsson went on to have a hearing aid implanted into his skull, again using titanium. Photographs of him around the time of that second operation show him grinning with delight and, in the process, confidently exposing his upper teeth.

Professor Brånemark did not immediately publicise his results with osseointegrated implants, as he was acutely aware that the history of implanted teeth replacements was one of poor science, vulnerable patients, false promises and failure. Additionally, orthodox dentistry at this time concentrated on disease prevention and the preservation of teeth and gum tissues. Given the disastrous results to date, experimentation with implants was frowned upon.

'Most of the conventionally used implants behave unpredictably and will eventually fail,' was how Professor George Zarb, a distinguished Canadian dental researcher, summed it up at the time. 'Most reported implant techniques do not survive scientific scrutiny.'

Because implants were suspect, the majority of dental schools did little more than mention the scientific facts surrounding implants. They did not go into the details. What would have been the point? It was an area of dentistry where only frauds and the foolhardy would go. Where the frauds and the foolhardy went, misery followed. Elaine Williams-McClarence's book, *A Matter Of Balance*, provides an in-depth and insightful history of osseointegration and the remarkable work of Brånemark. According to her: 'The older implant technologies often left a patient with worse dental problems after their surgery than before. It was this,' she wrote, 'that led to the majority of the dental profession regarding all implant techniques with scorn.'

All this meant that, by the time Brånemark discovered that titanium could be accepted by and integrated into bone, any positive results he achieved were likely to be greeted with scepticism. With the negative aura surrounding everything to do with implants he decided that experimentation should be carried out discreetly and successes should be recorded rather than trumpeted. Nonetheless, small stories crept out now and again and appeared in newspapers.

One of them caught the eye of a renowned opera singer named Olle Bohlin from Gothenburg. Bohlin was in such trouble with his teeth that he concluded he would have to learn to do something else, since continuing to go on stage and to open his troublesome mouth was beginning to fade as a career option. Not to mention the fact that, because eating was causing painful ulcers in his mouth, he had lost too much weight.

Bohlin decided that dental implants would be the solution to his problems and asked Brånemark to accept him as a patient in the early days, after Gosta Larsson. After his treatment, the opera singer was ecstatic. He could act and sing with confidence and, having not enjoyed food for more than a decade, he was able to chew with comfort and quickly regained the lost weight. Inevitably, he spoke publicly about the transformative medical treatment he had received. This may have surprised the team doing the implants because for several centuries those who had lost their teeth and became dental amputees didn't want anyone to know about it. Many of them became socially reclusive and those who managed with false teeth were rarely enthusiastic enough about their dentures to want to promote the denture-wearing experience in public. Implants were quite different. Once they got used to them, patients actively wanted to talk about them.

The problems that led people to Brånemark varied widely. The first half dozen patients included: Larsson, who had been crippled by a malformed mouth; Bohlin, who, having lost a lot of his teeth, had been fitted with unsuccessful bridgework that resulted in cysts forming in his jaw and consequent eating problems; and a young man who was missing not just his front teeth but part of his jawbone as a result of connecting facially with a golf club swung with vigour by a pal during horseplay. In this particular case, Brånemark's team grafted bone from the patient's hip on to his jaw before embarking on the rest of the implant process. Again, the operation was a success.

What is fascinating about Brånemark's approach was that, from the beginning, he didn't look for, or work on, easy cases, although this would have been the simplest and quickest way to publicise the phenomenal success of titanium implants. He wanted to test the components under the most extreme conditions, rather than under the best possible circumstances. So he and his team undertook the treatment of people who suffered from ectodermal dysplasia, a congenital condition where the patient never develops any teeth at all. They treated patients suffering from cleft palate and patients who had lost all their teeth. They even treated patients who, in addition to having lost their teeth, had lost substantial amounts of bone as a result of wearing dentures for many decades. By virtue of taking on the cases with the worst prognoses and the worst problems, they developed a two-step approach to dental implants which was repeated, successfully, again and again.

The first step in that two-step process was to prepare a precisely measured site in the jawbone into which an implant could be inserted. The implant would then be left alone for a period of time to ensure that the bone embraced this strange new arrival and grew around and into it, thereby rendering it secure.

It sounds simple enough but simple it is not. First of all, treatment had to be carried out under sterile conditions, more akin to those prevailing in orthopaedic surgery than in a dental practice. The delicate interior of bone has to be handled carefully during surgery to reduce the amount of damage caused.

The team learned as they went along: one of the key factors they discovered was that the interior of bone is extremely sensitive to temperatures above 42°C. This critical temperature can easily be exceeded, using regular high-speed dental drills. When such high temperatures are applied to bone, even for a short period, they can compromise the capacity of bone to form a secure biological bond with titanium and result in an implant failure. Clearly, any variation in temperature at the site of the surgery needed to be tightly controlled. This was achieved by the use of specially designed, low-speed drills. Additionally, a series of drills was used that ensured a gentle and gradual widening of the implant site and at all times during use they were kept cool by applying a constant stream of saline solution.

When the implant had firmly integrated with the jawbone the next step was to attach a post, called an 'abutment', on to which the replacement tooth would be attached. These posts projected up through the gum and provided a secure foundation to which to attach replacement teeth. Once small gold screws attached these final components, patients received a fixed set of teeth that did not rest on the gum and were not removable by the patient. This was in strong contrast to a complete plastic denture that had to be removed for cleaning, could become ill fitting, shifting and causing painful ulcers, and could even fall out unannounced at unexpected times. Patients could bite into the hardest apple or the thickest steak. They could smile. They could swim underwater. They could now sing, laugh and talk with confidence.

Brånemark was delighted with the results but he understood that he faced a broader and in some ways a more difficult challenge. A complete surgical protocol, including instrumentation and techniques, needed to be developed to ensure that other surgical teams could emulate this clinical success. This was accomplished in collaboration with his innovative surgical nurse, who has requested that she be referred to simply as 'Barbro' in this book. Brånemark also needed to build up a track record, quietly and without fuss. This could be achieved only by a careful study that would withstand close scientific scrutiny. Such a study would require meticulous document-ation of each case, recording not only success but failures and complications over time, as well as a rigorous statistical presentation of the results. Brånemark and his team waited for ten years before they published results that showed a success rate of more than 90 per cent in both upper and lower jaws.

Twenty-five years after the first implants, Sweden's excellent patient care record system showed that 95 per cent of implants going into the upper jaw had succeeded, as had more than 98 per cent of those going into the lower jaw. The lower rate of success for the upper jaw is a result of the more porous quality of the bone and the presence of the maxillary sinuses. The sinuses are naturally occurring cavities within the cheekbone. They normally come to our attention only when they become filled up with fluid, as can occur in the painful condition of sinusitis, or as one of the symptoms produced by the common cold virus or some allergic conditions. When these cavities, which normally contain air, have fluid within them the resonance of the voice changes, giving rise to the characteristic nasal quality of someone with a cold. These cavities reduce the amount of bone available for implants in the upper jaw.

At this point, coming towards the end of the 20th century, a quarter century of success with implants could be contrasted with the disastrous implant experiments of the earlier part of the century. Roughly eighty thousand patients had been successfully treated in Sweden and word was spreading.

Initially Brånemark's achievements did arouse some opposition at home in Sweden. What was becoming known as the 'Gothenburg' method of dental implants (the name of the city where Brånemark was based) was not, despite the emerging statistics, universally accepted as a major and positive development. Traditionalists called it expensive, painful and dangerous. The supposed danger lay in the risk posed to the mouth's protection against infection by the invasion of the delicate oral tissues that was an essential part of the surgery. The authorities also weighed in against the innovator, ordering him to destroy several dogs into whose mouths implants had been inserted in the early stages of his work. Brånemark would not accept that there was any medical reason for putting down animals that had virtually become pets of his team. The dogs, dead, would offer no additional evidence on implant surgery, whereas the dogs, kept alive, would continue to offer data. Eventually, the medical council gave up on it and allowed the dogs to live. All the dogs were extremely well cared for and lived out their natural life, lovingly looked after by members of the team.

Brånemark is not a man who suffers fools gladly. He responded with vigour and humour, making himself increasingly popular with those who admired his work and increasingly unpopular with those who thought him a high-tech charlatan. The latter group made personal attacks on him, the least offensive of which was to point out that he 'wasn't even a dentist'. True, the professor agreed. But he did train dentists and he was a medical doctor and a surgeon. His combative response to criticisms meant that universities were reluctant to support him, so he set up his own clinic, maintained by donations from industry. While opposition mounted, so did the numbers of successfully treated patients.

No matter how uniform the success and careful the methodology of Brånemark's studies, outside Sweden, the Gothenburg method met with even more scepticism than in the innovator's own country. Many dental surgeons and, more importantly, their patients, had been disappointed over and over again by previous attempts at implants and didn't want to know about yet another method, pioneered by a Swede they'd never heard of, using a metal nobody knew much about.

In America and Europe, the issue wasn't ignorance but hostility. To consider the issue of dental implants, given their grim history, seemed barely ethical to many dentists. Others had developed their own implant systems and societies formed to promote them. Most of these methods had been subjected to little or no scientific investigation and most amounted to human experimentation. It didn't help that some of the news gathered about the Swedish pioneer had appeared in publications like *Reader's Digest.* While such magazines were popular with readers, they were mostly viewed by medical professionals as being hotbeds of myth and medical misinformation. Published stories were often heavily coated with unjustified optimism, in turn giving rise to unrealistic expectations on the part of patients.

While Brånemark's research findings were often greeted with scepticism, a few medical professionals fell into Geoffrey Moore's category of 'early adopters', a term he developed in the context of the early high-tech industry in his book, *Crossing the Chasm* (1991). Such adopters are more visionary than the norm, seeing past the scepticism of the majority and recognising the important clinical possibilities of the procedure in question. One such person was Professor George

Zarb from Toronto, Canada who decided to visit Gothenburg and observe Brånemark's work at first hand. He was so impressed by what he saw that he decided to try and replicate the work in an independent study with his own patients in Toronto. He designed a rigorous scientific protocol and his results, which entirely replicated and validated Brånemark's work, were presented at the now famous Toronto Osseointegration Conference in 1982.

The tide turned. The independent replication study in North America had shown that dental implants *ad modum* Brånemark could work. From this time on the technique was no longer called the Gothenburg method but became known internationally as the 'Brånemark' method.

I first heard about Brånemark's work in 1982 as a result of this conference. To me, it had all the marks of a serious breakthrough, with the potential to solve the otherwise insoluble problems of the dental amputees who were my patients. I couldn't wait to meet the man and see at first hand precisely what he was doing.

By now Per-Ingvar Brånemark had managed to attract an international group of high-profile, authoritative supporters who were prepared to fight for his method. He called these his pioneer teams. They included teams in the Mayo Clinic, Rochester, the University of Toronto, the Catholic University of Leuven, and centres in Spokane, Washington, Texas, Paris, Sydney, Perth, Tokyo and Barcelona. We were honoured and delighted when he invited our own team in the Blackrock Clinic to be one of them. As well as myself as surgeon and an exceptionally talented surgical nurse, Bronagh Doran O'Reilly, the team consisted of two prosthodontists, Frank Houston from Trinity College Dublin Dental School and Gerard Buckley from Cork University Dental School. Shortly afterwards, Dr Michael Galvin and Dr Andrew Woolfe began to provide prosthodontic services to implant patients in Limerick and Dublin.

I placed the first Brånemark implants in Mount Carmel Hospital in Dublin in 1983, in a female patient who had lost all her lower teeth. They changed this woman's life and continue to function perfectly to

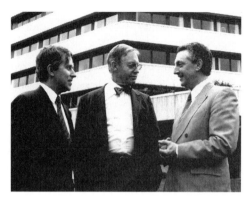

Fig. 7.2

this day. Just as the word had spread in Sweden and Canada, the word gradually spread in Ireland and elsewhere in Europe. A safe, proven and transformative surgery was now available to dental amputees.

Blackrock Clinic

We were especially privileged, as one of Professor Brånemark's pioneer teams, to enjoy a close and personal and professional working relationship with him in the newly opened Blackrock Clinic. Along with his nurse, Barbro, he operated with us pro bono on several Irish patients with serious congenital or acquired defects. He also provided international advanced teaching courses there that attracted surgeons from many different countries. Fig. 7.2 shows Professors Brånemark (centre), van Steenberghe and Harris in the Blackrock Clinic in 1986. In conjunction with Professor van Steenberghe in the University of Leuven and Professor Brånemark in the University of Gothenburg, our team in Blackrock Clinic became part of the European Osseo-integration Training Centre. This early close collaboration with Professor Brånemark in Blackrock Clinic made us very much part of the international movement in this emerging field and we have enjoyed this collaboration over the years to the present day.

Within a few years other Irish surgeons began placing implants and establishing their own teams. These early surgery adopters included Doctors Nicholas Mahon (RIP), Spencer Woolfe, Peter Cowan and Seán Sheridan. Today there are many well-trained specialist-led teams in Ireland offering implant services to a very high standard.

With the support of his pioneer teams and the kind of international collaboration Brånemark favoured, the story of dental implants shifted radically, worldwide. The innovator's insistence on careful documentation and meticulous scientific research, together with his resilience and resolve and the marvellous enthusiasm of successfully treated patients, made the outcome inevitable. Dental implants, which had traditionally been seen as based on disreputable human research, gradually became a scientifically proven and recognised procedure that would change and radically improve the lives of millions.

Professor Brånemark has received extensive international recognition for his work and contribution to dentistry from the highest institutions worldwide. This includes the awarding of an honorary fellowship of the Faculty of Dentistry in the Royal College of Surgeons in Ireland. His work extended outside the field of dentistry into the rehabilitation of major defects in the facial region, as well as orthopaedics and ENT surgery. These are outlined in the next chapter.

In the space of thirty years implant dentistry has radically changed the face of dentistry and the lives of millions. It has progressed from the activities of a handful of international pioneer teams to the mainstream of dental education and thousands of dental providers worldwide. This was all started by a man who was not even a dentist and who had been aiming at quite a different target when he began his ground-breaking research on blood circulation in rabbits.

8

Putting Dental Implants to Work

Modern osseointegrated titanium dental implants have achieved something that was once thought virtually impossible – the long-term function and survival of foreign implanted material within living bone. More than thirty years of careful patient follow-ups have confirmed that up to 98 per cent of these implants have the possibility of continuing to function successfully over a patient's lifetime. Although titanium implants are now used in different parts of the human body to help to restore and replace missing body parts or to restore function, their first proven application was in dentistry.

If you have been wearing conventional removable dentures and, as a result, found that your diet has become restricted or you have suffered badly from loss of appearance, confidence or self-esteem, an implants-supported prosthesis can transform your life. The following is an extract from a testimonial by M.W., a forty-two-year-old female patient who had lost all her upper and lower teeth, which were then restored by means of dental implants: It provides an insight into the positive impact dental implants can have on quality of life.

> I would like to take this opportunity to thank you for changing my life and giving me back my confidence. I will never forget the day I drove to see you, thinking to myself, what am I doing even considering having implants done and that I shouldn't spend this sort of money on myself. As you know I went through a very difficult separation and lost almost everything and here I was considering having implants done. I spent my life putting everyone and everything before myself and neglected my own

wellbeing. I had lost all my confidence and hated the fact that I had lost so many teeth and had to wear dentures. It's very difficult to explain to anyone how that feels. I couldn't eat properly and would avoid going to restaurants with friends. I even tried not to laugh or smile so that I wouldn't show my teeth. This is not the way to live your life…

My life has really changed for the better and I am always smiling now. It's amazing how free I feel and how I don't avoid photos or eating out.

Apart from the cosmetic side of things I no longer have pain or difficulty in eating certain foods. I love eating fruit and nuts and I don't even have to think about whether I can or not now. In fact I think my implants are even stronger than my own teeth.

I would highly recommend implants to any one who has dentures and not to wait for years to have them done.

My brother made a calendar for my mother for Christmas and put a photo of each family member on the date of their birthday and any other special occasion. He called me to see if I had any photos of me smiling as he had lots but I wasn't smiling in any of his. Guess what – neither did I!!! I can't wait for this year's calendar!

In this chapter, I'm going to take a look at the various clinical situations in which implants can be used to restore missing teeth. This account is, of necessity, somewhat technical and detailed but if you are considering having one or more dental implants, it may be helpful to you. I can deal only with general principles and it can never be overemphasised that every patient is unique and that only a careful clinical examination and assessment by a patient's own dentist can determine which treatment options are advisable or even possible. Before dealing with specific clinical applications it will be useful to clear up some common misconceptions about the role of dental implants.

First of all it should be appreciated that a dental implant is not a replacement for missing teeth. It functions more as a tooth root,

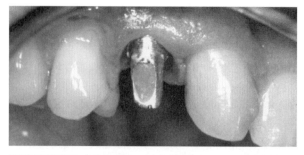

Fig. 8.1

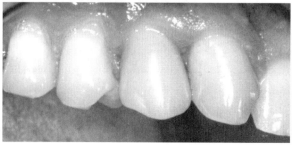

Fig. 8.2

the purpose of which is to provide a durable support on to which replacement teeth can be attached. Dentists use the term 'prosthesis' for the replacement tooth or teeth. As we will see, a prosthesis can take many forms: a crown, which is a single tooth attached to an implant; a bridge, in which two or more teeth are attached to as few as two implants; or a denture, which rests on or attaches to the implants. The prosthesis itself may be fixed to the implants and never removed by the patient or it may be a removable type of prosthesis. In the latter case it takes the form of a denture that, although attached firmly to the implants, will need to be removed for cleaning every day.

The following illustrates the process for a single missing tooth. A screw-shaped titanium implant is surgically placed within the jaw-bone and projects through the gum tissues. This part is known as an abutment (Fig. 8.1). Fig. 8.2 shows the final appearance when a crown (the fixed prosthesis) is made and attached to the abutment.

The second point that sometimes causes confusion is the fact that, when many teeth have been lost, it is not always necessary – or possible – to place an individual implant for every missing tooth. Using this approach a few implants can support many teeth.

The third important message is that it is always the prosthesis that replaces the missing teeth and not the implants. It is the prosthesis that the patient will see and feel in their mouth and the quality of the prosthesis that will determine whether a patient is happy with the outcome of the treatment. Although many patients will say that they would like to have implants, their wish is often based on what they imagine implants will do for them, usually give them the perfect teeth they have always wanted. Media promotions, advertisements and material sourced on the internet can give rise to misleading expectations of what can be achieved. Hence careful examination, visualisation of the end result and appropriate planning of implant treatment are essential if disappointments are to be avoided. When a patient has complex or difficult problems it is often advisable to consult with specialists from two different fields: the surgeon who will place the implants and the prosthodontist who will construct and fit the teeth.

With these points in mind we can look at some of the more common situations in which implants may be of benefit.

When all the lower and/or upper teeth are missing

These were the first applications that Brånemark and his team developed for clinical practice. Prior to this time the treatment of patients who had lost all their teeth had remained virtually unchanged since the introduction of the complete removable denture – with all the limitations and accompanying functional, psychological and aesthetic problems already discussed.

Fig. 8.3 and Fig. 8.4 shows how five implants can be used to provide support for a fixed-bridge prosthesis of approximately twenty teeth.

It can be seen that in this situation there are fewer implants than teeth and the implants appear to be placed close together towards the front of the jaw. The reason for this is twofold. Firstly, the bone shrinkage that follows the loss of all teeth means that there is much less space available for implants. Secondly, towards the back and side of

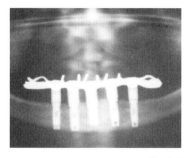

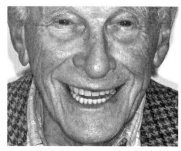

Fig. 8.3

Fig. 8.4

the mouth, there is a large nerve that runs through the lower jawbone on each side. This is responsible for providing sensation in the region of the lip and chin. In people who still have most of their teeth the nerve lies deep within the bone. As a result of the bone shrinkage that naturally occurs when all teeth have been lost, this nerve comes to lie up close to the surface. The nerve itself has not moved but the bone above it that held the teeth is lost and this accounts for the more superficial position of the nerve in the remaining bone.

Because of this, in most cases in which all the teeth have been lost, there would be a real danger of damaging this nerve if implants were placed above it. Fortunately the main trunk of the nerve does not travel all the way forward through the jaw. Its position can be seen on x-ray, where it appears as a translucent line about an eighth of an inch wide (Fig. 8.5). Once the nerve has been clearly identified, in the vast majority of patients there is room to place implants safely towards the front of the jaw. In order to provide teeth further back in the mouth the part of the prosthesis carrying the premolar or molar teeth projects backwards from the last implant.

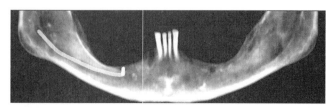

Fig. 8.5

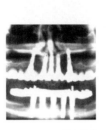

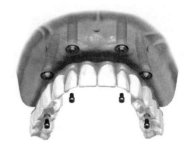

Fig. 8.6   Fig. 8.7

Without a doubt, the treatment of the lower jaw with implants in this way has had the best track record of all implant applications to date with regard to longevity, the absence of serious complications, ease of maintenance and patient satisfaction with function, speech and appearance.

When all the upper teeth are to be replaced Brånemark advised the use of four to six implants to provide support for a fixed prosthesis (Fig. 8.6). For a number of reasons, the replacement of upper teeth with implants is technically somewhat more problematic than replacing teeth in the lower jaw (Fig. 8.7).

Firstly, the upper jaw does not consist of solid bone throughout – there are natural cavities within it. These cavities consist of the sinuses on each side and the nose towards the centre. As these natural cavities do not contain any bone, they can limit the space available for implant placement.

Fig. 8.8 shows an x-ray of the typical appearance of someone who has lost all their upper teeth, with the natural sinus and nasal cavities labelled. These appear black on x-ray, as the absence of bone allows the x-rays to pass through. The restricted area of bone that might be available for implants is denser and appears grey underneath.

This reduction in the available bone area may preclude the placement of sufficient implants to provide a fixed prosthesis, particularly if the remaining bone has become very thin as a result of shrinkage. The normal two-dimensional panoramic x-ray shows the natural

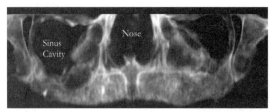

Fig. 8.8

cavities but does not provide any information about the thickness or width of the remaining bone. In order to do an accurate assessment of the quantity of bone, a CT scan may be necessary. This type of scan provides a three-dimensional view of the upper jaw and allows for accurate measurements to be obtained.

Planning treatment in this way allows the patient and surgeon to gain a better understanding of what might be achieved and, more importantly, to identify any limitations and problems that are likely to be encountered. The identification of any difficulties at this early stage is vitally important so that measures may be taken to ensure that the patient obtains a predictable result. The good news is that it's nearly always possible to overcome the problem of insufficient bone. But I'll come to that in due course.

Another issue that often needs to be addressed in the case of upper-teeth replacement is to ensure that the prosthesis provided is satisfactory from the patient's point of view. Problems can arise as a result of the pattern of bone shrinkage. For example in the upper jaw the bone tends to shrink from the outermost part, where it lies against the cheeks and lips, in an inward direction towards the roof of the mouth. Implants placed in such bone may now lie too far inward for the teeth that are to be attached. Ideally, they need to be nearer the cheek. In order to overcome this discrepancy between the ideal teeth and implant positions and the reality of what is available, it may be necessary to compensate by making the prosthesis bulkier or thicker. As a result it may become very difficult to construct a fixed prosthesis that does not unduly interfere with speech, provides adequate support for the upper lip and overcomes the flattened appearance that so readily identifies a denture wearer with advanced bone shrinkage.

Once again this problem must be assessed in advance with the correct detailed clinical and x-ray investigations. I say 'must', because once the implants have been placed there is really very little that can be done about their position and this can lead to disappointment on the part of the patient. If the limitations are detected in advance the possibility of correcting the condition by measures such as increasing the amount of bone available for implants can be considered. The procedure by which missing bone can be replaced is known as bone augmentation.

Another possibility in such situations is to consider a removable overdenture, which often gives more flexibility with tooth positioning and support for facial tissues. Studies have shown that patients adapt extremely well to a removable upper overdenture, which may allow them to achieve better phonetics and better hygiene procedures than a fixed prosthesis.

Removable prosthesis or overdenture

An overdenture, which is removable by the patient, is nearly always an option when all the upper teeth are missing, provided sufficient implants can be placed to support it. It consists of a denture that attaches to the implants by means of clips or other attachments (Fig. 8.9, Fig. 8.10 and Fig. 8.11).

Sometimes patients will be disappointed when first presented with the idea of having a removable denture component in combination with implants. Initially they may not appreciate the very significant

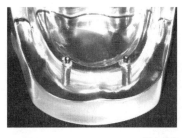

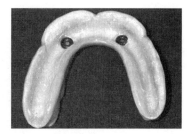

Fig. 8.9   Fig. 8.10

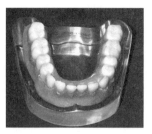

Fig. 8.11

advantages an implant-supported overdenture will offer, as compared to regular complete dentures. The majority of patients who choose this option find that they are extremely happy with the end result.

Overdentures on implants can overcome many significant and worrying problems that bother people who have to wear top and bottom dentures. Those problems, which surface almost every day, include loose dentures that drop, shift and move about, difficulty in chewing, pain and ulceration in the soft tissues of the mouth on which the dentures rest and the poor appearance that typifies the long-term denture wearer.

It is possible to eliminate many of those problems by attaching an overdenture to rigid implants. The secure attachment provides a high level of retention, stability and security during eating and talking. There is little danger that the overdenture will pop out unexpectedly. When patients chew with an overdenture they will be able to exert significantly more chewing force than they could with dentures, as the overdenture won't become displaced. Nor will it dig into the soft tissues because that kind of movement will be resisted by the implants.

This may read as if overdentures attached to implants simply prevent some of the discomforts and disasters associated with ordinary dentures. In fact, the end results are a lot more positive than just disaster prevention. For example, any previous restrictions on diet will be significantly lessened. As the retention of the overdentures is so much improved, it allows the dentist, where necessary, to increase their bulk and offset the position of the teeth to establish the most favourable appearance. This flexibility also allows the dentist to restore the support or vertical dimension of the face and, as a result, achieve a much more pleasing appearance. Restoring the vertical dimension can be a great aid to overcoming problems with sibilant speech that are sometimes obvious in denture wearers, especially when they are talking over a microphone. This is a particularly high priority for radio or television presenters or for anyone else who speaks for a living.

Overdentures on implants also feel different because the loads applied to the implants during function partially transmit sensation into the jawbone, as real teeth do. This is known as proprioception. Patients find that they can appreciate the texture of foods in a way that is quite different from when they wear normal complete dentures.

There are, however a number of disadvantages to wearing an over-denture retained by implants. These relate to the way that the over-denture attaches to the implants. Such attachments can be made of metal clips or bars, rubber O-rings, nylon insets or magnets. All tend to loosen and wear over time, as does the overdenture itself. Overdentures therefore need regular adjustment to maintain their retention, periodic replacement of attachments and relines or replacement of the dentures.

In Chapter 3 we looked at the problems caused by the continuous irreversible bone shrinkage that occurs when people wear normal removable dentures. One of the most important long-term benefits of implant-supported overdentures is that implants stimulate the bone and prevent such changes happening. In this way the problems that result from continuous bone shrinkage are virtually eliminated.

Although an overdenture can solve many problems when there is insufficient bone to support a complete prosthesis, there needs to be a certain minimum of bone available for all implants. Anyway, many people will prefer not to have a removable prosthesis and really want to have a fixed bridge of upper teeth that remains in place all the time.

In such situations, limitations in the amount of bone available can be overcome. Where bone is deficient it can be reconstructed by adding new bone and making it suitable for implant placement. This is called bone grafting or bone augmentation. If there is advanced bone loss in the upper jaw it is now also possible to place longer implants that will bypass the diminished jawbone. These are inserted into a dense bone in the cheek and are called 'zygomatic' implants.

Bone augmentation/grafting

There is nothing very new about grafting bone to the jaw. Before the availability of osseointegrated dental implants, bone grafting was used to try to build up sufficient bone to make wearing complete dentures possible. Although the bone graft itself was a success, in the sense that it was accepted and became incorporated into the patient's own bone, the procedure was a miserable failure. The reason for this is that, over time, the grafted bone suffered the same fate as the patient's original bone and rapidly underwent shrinkage, as the bone wasn't stimulated when the patient was wearing complete dentures. It was quite an extensive surgical procedure for something that produced only a short-term improvement. However, when Professor Brånemark combined his implants with a bone graft, he obtained a completely different result. The presence of the implants provided a loading stimulus to the newly formed bone and, as we have seen, when bone is subject to functional loads it strengthens and does not shrink. Once again, meticulous follow-up of patients demonstrated that the presence of the implants within the newly reconstructed bone ensured its long-term survival.

Sometimes the graft is obtained from elsewhere in the body of the patient who is to receive it. This, known as an 'autogenous' bone graft, has traditionally been considered the gold standard. It is worth spending a moment to consider why it so highly regarded. Firstly, there is no possibility of the transmission of disease as the graft is drawn from the patient's own bone. Secondly, the patient will not reject the graft, as it is not a 'foreign tissue' from another person or species. Thirdly, because of these properties, it is not necessary to treat the graft with chemicals or radiation to render it sterile or prevent rejection.

The unprocessed autogenous graft is the patient's own living bone and still holds new bone-forming cells and growth-promoting hormones. This will ensure rapid incorporation into a patient's existing bone and encourage the formation of new bone.

The main drawback to an autogenous bone graft is that it requires the creation of a second surgical site to obtain it. This is known as the donor site. Sometimes, when only a small volume of graft material is required to treat a small bone defect, it can be obtained from within the mouth However when large amounts of bone are needed, as is often the case for an upper jaw that has undergone extensive bone loss, a donor site is required outside the mouth. A well-documented area for obtaining such bone is from the crest of the hipbone. With careful planning, many centres – including our own – have obtained excellent long-term results using bone from this area.

However autogenous bone grafts have considerable drawbacks that need to be taken into consideration. The necessity for a second surgical donor site can make the procedure more complex, especially when extensive grafts need to be obtained. The harvesting of the graft from some donor sites may require more advanced surgical training and, for the patient, a general anaesthetic and admission into hospital. The donor surgical site is subject to its own complications and problems in the post-operative period.

Practitioners should discuss this whole procedure fully with patients so that they understand and accept any risk involved. In this regard it is worth remembering that there is no such thing as surgery that is entirely free of risk. Even the simple removal of a tooth can on occasion lead to serious problems in the post-operative period. Strict protocols for achieving good results mean that the technique of bone grafting is very demanding. If it is not carried out correctly, bone loss can occur very rapidly and the soft tissues overlying the graft can be difficult to handle.

Because of the drawbacks of autogenous bone grafts other types of graft material have been developed that can be obtained commercially.

'Xenografts', or bone mineral, consist of bone obtained from other animals such as cows. The bone is subjected to harsh chemical treatment with an alkaline agent that removes any protein content and is then sterilised to remove any infective agents. Because all the protein has been removed there is no danger of transmitting a prion disease such as CJD, which is the human variant of bovine encephalitis – more commonly known as 'mad cow disease'. Likewise, the absence of proteins means it will not stimulate a rejection process in the person receiving it. The resulting bone mineral is devoid of any living cells or bone growth factors and is really an inert calcium scaffold. Fig. 8.12 shows its appearance under a microscope. The islands of inert bone, which are lighter in colour, are seen within living bone that appears darker in colour. The bone mineral will, however, rapidly become incorporated into a patient's own bone and, over time, allow new bone to grow into it. It is not as readily resorbed by the body as autogenous bone and takes longer to shrink away.

The advantages of a xenograft are clear. There is no need for a second operation at another surgical site with its associated incon-venience and possible complications. Properly treated xenografts are not rejected but are incorporated well into existing bone. As far as has been ascertained, the procedure is completely safe and has been fully cleared for use in the United States and Europe. Most of the leading universities and centres involved in this work worldwide, including those in Ireland, use it. The author has also had it used as the material of choice in his own mouth.

The drawback of xenograft bone mineral is that it must be used carefully within specified protocols that limit its usefulness, especially for large grafts. It is the author's opinion that in its present form it is not suitable for patients who need large grafts for an upper jaw that has

Fig. 8.12

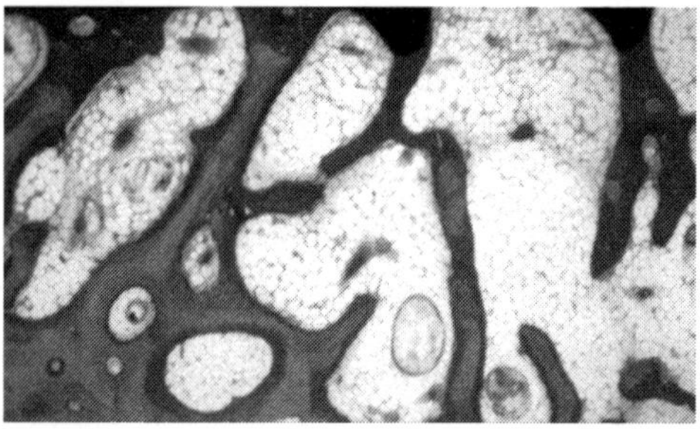

undergone advanced bone loss. It is sometimes mixed with autogenous bone to increase the bulk of material available and is the treatment of choice for small localised bone grafting and, as we will see, when grafting into the sinus.

One of the main drawbacks of xenografts is their lack of growth-promoting agents and other stimulating factors that help new bone to form, as these have been removed in the processing. Promising research into combining the mineral with genetically produced growth factors suggest that we are on the way to a wider range of situations in which xenografts can successfully be used. However, it should be stressed that much of this is early research, with only a small number of clinical applications.

Another type of graft material available is a 'homograft', cadaver bone obtained from other human beings. This bone is demineralised to remove all the calcium and often freeze-dried and sterilised. It is popular within the United States but not so much in Europe. The main advantage is that it appears to retain some growth-hormone activity and those who use it report excellent results.

The main drawback of homograft material is the possibility of the presence of prions and of disease transmission, as there have been instances of disease transmission from other cadaver-obtained grafts. Although it is accepted that the risk is very low, most of the centres of excellence in Europe and indeed in the US choose instead to use autografts or xenografts. At our own centre we made a decision to not use this material, as I would not have it placed it in the mouth of family members or in my own mouth.

Sinus bone augmentation

When missing upper teeth towards the side and back of the mouth are being replaced, the lack of bone beneath the sinus may prevent implants from being successfully placed. Sometimes it is possible to place a graft within the sinus, beneath the sinus membrane, using xenograft bone mineral. Before carrying out this procedure it is essential to ensure that there are no pre-existing sinus problems or altered anatomy that might interfere with success or cause complications. The author's view is that this is best achieved by obtaining a CT scan that includes a view of the sinus so it can be established that it is free of disease and is likely to have satisfactory drainage. If disease is discovered, consultation with an ENT surgeon may be required to clear the condition before sinus lift surgery is undertaken. Fig. 8.13 shows a sinus with little bone available for implants. The increased bone has been obtained by means of a sinus augmentation carried out at the time the implants were placed. The final result with bridgework in place can be seen in Fig. 8.14.

Replacement of teeth when the patient retains many teeth of their own

When only a few teeth are to be replaced, using implants needs to be carefully weighed against other options that are available, such as bridgework. In the case of a single missing tooth, a crown supported by an implant is the treatment of choice, providing that good bone

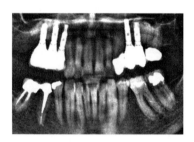

Fig. 8.13

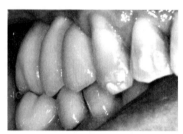

Fig. 8.14

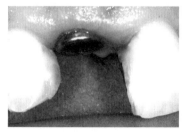

Fig. 8.15

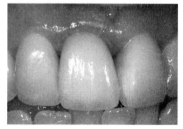

Fig. 8.16

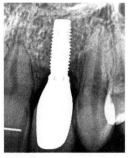
Fig. 8.17

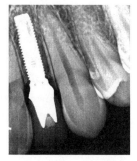
Fig. 8.18

volume and suitable gum tissue are available. This is shown in Fig. 8.15 and Fig. 8.16, demonstrating that the demands for a good appearance can be met. In a favourable situation this procedure can provide excellent long-term results, without interfering with the teeth on either side of the gap. Fig. 8.17 and Fig. 8.18 show implants used toward the front of the mouth. Similar results can be obtained when more than one tooth is missing (Fig. 19) and implants can be combined with crowns or veneers on a patient's own natural teeth (Fig. 20).

However it is not always possible to achieve aesthetically pleasing results, especially in patients who naturally have a high smile line (showing not only the full extent of their teeth but the gum over them). In such case, the technical demands are very high as it will be necessary to produce a natural appearance for the teeth on the implants, ensuring that they emerge from the gum tissues in a harmonious way, as well as matching the adjacent teeth in shape, position and hue. Bone and gum shrinkage can make this difficult to achieve. A very careful assessment of these patients is required and will probably include impressions for study casts of the patient's teeth. The end result should be shown in wax on these models (diagnostic wax-up) so that both the patient and dentist can visualise it in advance. Sometimes preliminary procedures undertaken before or at the time the implants are placed, including bone grafts and/or grafts to the gum tissues, will be required in order to obtain a satisfactory outcome. In some cases, the patient may choose to accept a small cosmetic deficit rather than undergo these additional procedures. Again, a careful assessment is essential, which may take several visits to complete, and a team approach involving a number of specialists may be necessary in complex cases. If teeth have already drifted out of position they may need to be realigned before implant treatment begins.

One essential when treating patients who have retained some natural teeth is to ensure that any existing disease in the teeth and gums has been successfully treated prior to implant treatment. Although teeth are sometimes thought of as inert tissues lying in bone they are very much living structures, as anyone who has had toothache or extreme sensitivity to cold will attest. They are also attached to bone by a ligament that has significant defence mechanisms. Natural teeth can fight off infections but the downside is that infective gum disease may progress slowly over many years. When this is present, some nasty organisms can grow in the gum pockets that develop around the teeth.

Implants are inert metallic structures and cannot resist infection in the same way as natural teeth. If implants are placed in mouths with an existing infection there is a high likelihood that this will rapidly spread to the implants, with disastrous results. For this reason all infective processes must be cleared up in advance. This includes treating gum disease and removing any abscesses associated with existing teeth. Patients must accept responsibility for maintaining the health of the gum tissue around their natural teeth and implants, keeping a regular schedule with a dental hygienist who can provide ongoing advice and

Fig. 8.19

© *Professor David Harris: reproduced with patient's permission.*

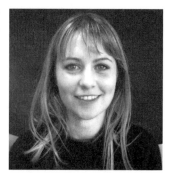

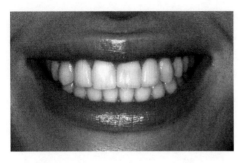

Fig. 8.20

help monitor and maintain oral hygiene.

In this chapter I have tried to give an insight into the most common situations that arise in relation to implants and some of the problems that may occur, emphasising the necessity for detailed assessment and planning as well as visualisation of the end result before treatment is begun. Good planning means working backwards from the desired end result and developing an individual treatment strategy for achieving it. In complex cases a team consisting of a specialist prosthodontist, who will plan and visualise the end result, and a specialist oral surgeon or periodontist to assess and carry out the surgical procedures will ensure the best result for the treatment.

In the early days of dental implants this approach was often reversed, with the emphasis on placing implants first, then working out how the teeth should be made. It soon became obvious that this was a shortsighted approach that could lead to successful implant placement but a very unhappy patient. It is essential that the dental team fully understand the patient's expectations. It is equally important that patients understand, before they embark on complex treatment, exactly what can be achieved, the limitations of the treatment and their own role and responsibilities in ensuring a successful outcome.

9

Advances in Implant Dentistry

The excellent results achieved by osseointegrated dental implants were at first greeted sceptically by the dental profession. This was understandable, as they had seen so many previous claims to success with dental implants end in disaster. Over a period of ten years or so, the new implants gradually became accepted by the wider dental profession and teaching institutes worldwide. Partly fuelled by patient demand and partly by companies that manufactured dental implants, which were quick to recognise a new market opportunity, there followed an era of increasingly focused research. There was intense curiosity about why implants managed to join to bone and become accepted as a body part rather than being rejected as a foreign body.

Academic teaching institutions also recognised that significant funding might be available for this area of research. Particular interest developed, not only in documenting success rates scientifically, but in looking at the cause and treatment of complications and problems that might occur. In addition, research was carried out to see how treatments might be improved and to widen the scope of possible clinical procedures. At the same time, there was a growing realisation of the need to improve both the aesthetics and patient acceptance of the results that could be obtained with implants.

The manufacturing companies in particular were keen to develop and simplify treatment, not least because they were convinced that patient demand would increase if the clinical process could be speeded up. The original treatment process, known as the 'delayed loading protocol', required three different stages with intervals between them to ensure that osseointegration took place and is shown in Fig. 9.1.

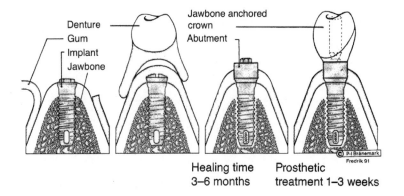

Healing time
3–6 months

Prosthetic
treatment 1–3 weeks

Fig. 9.1

Professor P.-I. Brånemark: permission of Nobel Biocare.

The reason for the waiting period after implant insertion was to allow sufficient healing time for the implants and for implants and bone to develop a strong, durable bond. This meant that the construction of replacement teeth could not even begin for a period of three months in the case of the lower jaw and six months for the upper. From the time the implants were in place a patient could wait up to nine months before they had their new teeth, during which time they had to continue wearing dentures. When bone grafting was involved the total treatment time could stretch to eighteen months.

This became the standard protocol for successful treatment and was based on the concept that no loads (e.g. chewing) should be placed on the implants until new bone had formed around them. Clearly this delay was not what patients wanted, although they accepted that it was necessary. When attempts were made to shorten this period of time, failures occurred.

Implant companies were keen to overcome these limitations by developing different designs and surfaces for their implants, in the hope that bone might join to them more quickly.

The first implants used by Brånemark were machined from pure titanium blocks. Early experiments to speed up the process involved modifying the design and also the surface of the implant, making it rougher in order to increase the surface area that would be in contact with bone. Many of these designs proved to be disastrous. Some companies coated the surface with a ceramic-like material that had been shown in experiments to join faster to bone. When these implants were placed in patients the new surface was found to separate from the implants. Many of the pioneers in the field became concerned about the undisciplined trial-and-error techniques being undertaken. There was concern that it might bring the whole area into disrepute and undo the success of the work carried out by Brånemark and his meticulous research.

Over time, however, research identified the optimum range of roughness for implant surfaces and various surface treatments that would improve the rate at which bone would grow on to implants without jeopardising the results. Today, many different manufacturers produce implants that can be expected to give good results.

Although faster bone growth on modern implants is a reality, Mother Nature will not be rushed and still demands time for new bone to form. The original treatment waiting time has been reduced to as little as six weeks but in order for procedures such as this to be successful much depends on the clinical findings for the individual patient. This has become known as the 'early loading protocol'.

Other research into the way implants function and how they may be protected from overloading during the critical healing period has led to specific clinical developments that allow replacement teeth to be fitted on the day the implants are placed. This is known as the 'immediate loading protocol'.

Teeth in a day, 1998 (Same-day teeth, Nobel Biocare)

Professor Brånemark brought his meticulous research skills to bear on these issues and in 1998 provided the first well-documented results for a technique he called 'Brånemark Novum' but which quickly came to be called 'same-day teeth'.

This technique took implant replacements to a new level. Patients who had lost all their teeth could attend in the morning for implant surgery and leave the same day with their new teeth (fixed bridgework) in place. This was a remarkable achievement and one that patients really appreciated. With his customary caution, Brånemark did not make the components and system for this protocol available commercially until a number of pioneer teams throughout the world had tested and carefully documented the technique on at least twenty patients in each centre to ensure that the outstanding results he had reported could be reliably replicated. No contact was permitted between the different teams and each documented its experience independently. Our own unit in the Blackrock Clinic, where I collaborated with Dr Ada Foster and Michael Doherty, was one of the participating centres. The teams' experiences were subsequently combined and published in 2001 as a textbook entitled *The Brånemark Novum Protocol for Same-Day Teeth*.

There was a remarkable degree of consensus among all the participating centres: the outstanding factor that emerged was the enthusiasm of patients who, for the first time, knew they could attend the clinic that morning and leave with their new teeth in place. Some of these early patients had had no teeth for twenty years or more. They became very emotional and even tearful when they found they had realised their dream and had 'their teeth back again'.

The key to this technique was the use of prefabricated components (Fig. 9.2), along with special surgical guides and implants that would allow them to be placed very precisely in position. The fact that the position could be so exactly predicted allowed the prefabricated

Fig. 9.2

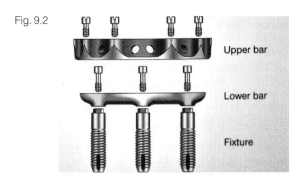

Upper bar

Lower bar

Fixture

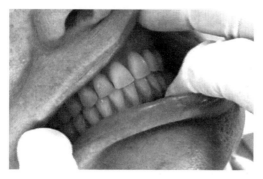
Fig. 9.3

bridgework to be accurately attached).

Same-day teeth attracted significant media interest worldwide and we were invited to demonstrate the technique on *The Richard and Judy Show* on ITV in December 1999. The programme team followed a patient attending the Blackrock Clinic on the day of treatment and then interviewed her in the studio some three months later (Fig. 9.3). The programme may be viewed on our website: www. blackrockclinicdental.ie.

Computer-assisted surgery and 3-D planning

One of the most exciting developments in implant dentistry over recent years has been the availability of CT scans and computer programs that allow an accurate three-dimensional model of the jawbones to be created. These programs allow for very clear identification and location of important anatomical structures such as nerves and sinus cavities. The accuracy of the measurements obtained far exceeds what can be achieved using normal x-rays. On a computer screen the 3-D model can be rotated in any direction and prospective implant sites viewed from any angle.

Some programs also include a library of different implants, any of which can be placed and manipulated within the screen model. In this way, trial implant surgery can now be planned in virtual reality on the computer, while teeth specially selected for a patient, together with information on the position in the mouth that will provide the best and most pleasing result, can also be also be scanned and integrated

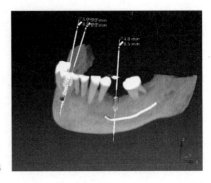

Fig. 9.4

into the 3-D model (Fig. 9.4). This all happens before patients undergo any treatment. The on-screen simulations let them appreciate the proposed end result and allow for any desired modifications. The surgeon can now confidently plan with great accuracy. The implant positions can be determined on screen and manoeuvred to ensure that they are placed as near as possible to the optimum position for the teeth that are to be attached.

Teeth in an Hour and minimally invasive surgery

The availability of this technology has clearly taken the Brånemark Novum technique one stage further. The process that allows such accurate transfer of planning to the surgical procedure is based on research carried out in the Catholic University of Leuven in Belgium by Professor Daniel van Steenberghe and his team. Our own centre has had the privilege of a close collaboration with this institution for more than twenty-five years. Professor van Steenberghe's contribution to the field received recognition in 2002 when he was inducted as an Honorary Fellow of the Faculty of Dentistry of the Royal College of Surgeons in Ireland.

Teeth in an Hour takes this technology even further and allows for the production of the replacement teeth in advance of surgery. This is achieved by downloading data from the scan, together with the planning information, directly to a specialised centre (Fig. 9.5 and Fig. 9.6). The data then moves from virtual reality to actual reality and is processed into a physical replica model. A specialised dental

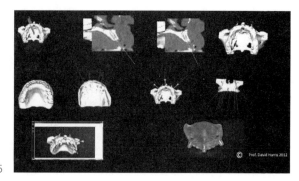

Fig. 9.5

laboratory can now process the replacement teeth originally designed for the patient as well as a special surgical guide. Fig. 9.7 shows Glen McEvoy of Eurocast Laboratories, Dublin, and Fig. 9.8 shows the completed prosthesis. With a preformed bridge of teeth and a surgical guide based on the virtual planning, the procedure can now be undertaken using minimally invasive surgery and, remarkably, the whole procedure for a patient with no teeth can be completed in less than an hour.

The use of minimally invasive surgery is a major medical advance. Normally during surgery the full area that is to be operated on has to be viewed, something that requires extensive surgical exposure. With minimally invasive (sometimes called keyhole) surgery, the whole procedure is carried out through a very small incision. It is normally performed via small cameras that allow the surgical site to be viewed or, as is the case for teeth in an hour, by accurately designed surgical

Fig. 9.7

Fig. 9.6

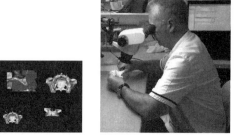

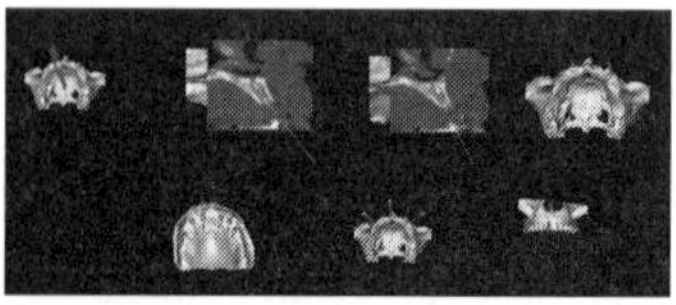

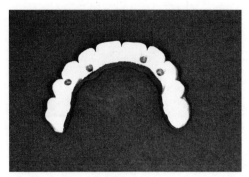

Fig. 9.8

guides. The advantages for the patient are that minimally invasive surgery eliminates the need for a wide surgical exposure and results in greatly reduced postoperative swelling and discomfort. Because of the keyhole incision, stitches are not normally required. The technique differs in one important way from keyhole surgery in medicine. It relies entirely on the surgical guides to ensure the correct position of the implants, whereas in medical use cameras, lenses or x-rays allow direct vision throughout the procedure. These templates are made on the basis of the computerised design provided by the surgeon and the correct transfer of information to the surgical site.

The bridgework produced in advance of the implants being placed is custom-designed for the patient to provide the best appearance, function, ease of cleaning and maintenance. Once again, although considerable work has to be carried out prior to the implant surgery, the real magic is that the patient attends for placement of the implants and leaves one hour later with the new teeth (fixed bridgework) in place.

The same computerised planning is used for zygomatic implants, which are explained in more detail in the following pages. These are used to replace missing teeth in the upper jaw when bone loss has become so severe that patients have insufficient remaining bone in which to place normal implants. Patients such as these suffer severe functional and psychological deficits and cannot manage to wear any kind of denture successfully. Computer-assisted planning, along with zygomatic implants, allows a temporary bridge to be completed within

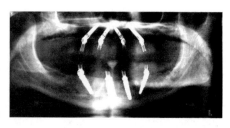

Fig. 9.9

one day of implant placement. Once again, the patient attending knows that there will be a rapid transition from having to put up with an impossible-to-wear upper denture to teeth that are fixed in place.

Teeth in a Day 2014

Further advances in providing Teeth in a Day have been facilitated by emerging long-term studies showing that as few as four implants can be used to provide a full bridge of teeth that are fixed to the implants on the same day. Fig. 9.9 shows four implants in each jaw that were used to support bridgework replacing missing upper and lower teeth. This technique has radically simplified the process for treating patients who have lost all their teeth and consequently reduced the cost of the providing this service. Although the technical and surgical costs are reduced, there is an added need for careful assessments and, in the author's opinion, a greater degree of surgical experience and prosthodontic skills is required to achieve a predictable outcome.

Zygomatic implants

When bone loss has progressed to the point when there is hardly any upper-jaw bone remaining, it may become impossible for a patient to function with any kind of upper denture. Even worse, the diminished bone remaining will often be insufficient to have regular dental implants inserted. Although extensive bone grafts from the hip can be used to overcome this problem this involves several surgeries and about eighteen months of treatment to complete. During this time the patient has to manage with a makeshift denture. 'Zygomatic' implants offer the possibility of removing the necessity for extensive bone grafting and a fixed prosthesis can be provided within twenty-four hours. Once again Professor Brånemark pioneered this technique and the long-term outcomes are proving very successful.

The zygomatic bone lies above the upper jaw and the sinuses within the cheek. It is readily accessible through the mouth and especially designed long implants can be surgically placed. Fig. 9.10 and Fig. 9.11 show the computerised planning and x-ray of zygomatic implants placed in a patient who had insufficient bone remaining for regular dental implants. These four implants were sufficient to support a fixed bridge of upper teeth. All the surgery is first visualised, planned and carried out in virtual reality on a special computer program.

Zygomatic implants have a number of advantages for a patient, as compared to bone grafting. Firstly, no second donor site is required. Secondly, the patient can have a fixed prosthesis fitted within twenty-four hours instead of having to wait for up to twelve to eighteen months for their teeth, as is often required with large bone grafts.

Over the past ten years the technique for using zygomatic implants has become well developed and refined. Although the

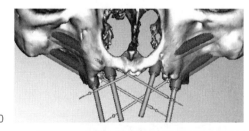

Fig. 9.10

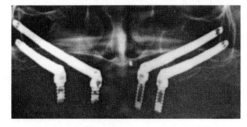

Fig. 9.11

surgery is significantly more extensive than that required for regular implants, the results can be excellent. For patients who have lost all their upper teeth and undergone severe bone shrinkage it has, in the author's opinion, become the treatment of choice, replacing large bone-grafting procedures. In association with Professor Leo Stassen consultant oral and maxillofacial surgeon in St James's Hospital, Dublin, Dr Frank Houston of the Dental School in Trinity College Dublin and Professor Malavez of the University of Brussels, we commenced a programme of providing these implants to support fixed bridgework in the Blackrock Clinic in 2008. In the same year Professor Gerry Kearns, consultant oral and maxillofacial surgeon, in conjunction with prosthodontist Dr Eddie Cotter, began to use them to support removable overdentures.

Eyes, ears, nose and hearing

Professor Brånemark realised that the phenomenon of osseo-integration was not specific to jaw bone and that the capacity to gain long-term anchorage of titanium inserts in bone could be applied to other areas of rehabilitation. His multidisciplinary team in Gothenburg looked at other circumstances in which prosthesis was necessary to replaced lost tissue, such as an eye or a nose or an ear. Up to this point such prosthetic replacements had no firm anchorage to keep them in place and often relied on glues that could very easily come undone.

Soon the team produced implants based on the original dental design to attach prosthetic replacements in the craniofacial and other regions of the body. Such defects often arise from congenital conditions, following traumatic injuries or as a result of necessary surgery to treat cancerous growths. The results were startlingly good. In fact these procedures were life-changing for those patients as they effectively restored their self-confidence and self-esteem and ability to lead a normal social life. For those recovering from surgery they held out hope that became an important part of their rehabilitation.

The Maxillofacial Unit in St James's Hospital has a substantial

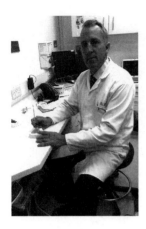

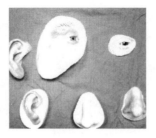

Fig. 9.13

Reproduced with kind permission of Niall Murphy.

Fig. 9.12

surgical programme in place to provide these procedures for the benefit of Irish patients. The prostheses that attach to the implants require the artistic and technical skills of a specially trained dental technician. These skills allow a silicone prosthesis to be produced that can blend in with the surrounding skin so as to be almost unnoticeable. The gifted Niall Murphy, chief maxillofacial technician, shown in Fig. 9.12, fulfils this important role in St. James's Hospital. Fig. 9.13 shows some examples of the types of prosthesis he produces. The patients involved gave their permission for their photographs be included in this book as they wished to ensure that other patients become aware that this treatment is available. Niall Murphy provided the prostheses.

Replacement ear

In the condition known as aural atresia the external ear fails to develop or does so in only a very rudimentary way. Plastic reconstructive surgeons have always acknowledged how difficult it is to reconstruct a missing ear that looks natural. Small implants attached to the bone on the side of the skull allow a specially constructed prosthesis (replacement ear) to be attached, producing an entirely natural appearance.

Fig. 9.14 shows a patient with two implants in place and Fig. 9.15 shows the prosthetic replacement for the ear securely attached.

This condition is particularly problematic in small children, as

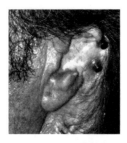
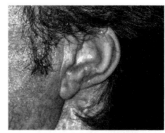

Fig. 9.14   Fig. 9.15

Reproduced with patient's permission.

children can be very cruel to one another when one of them looks different. A human side to this story is that the affected children sometimes went from being the taunted as a class oddity to becoming the amazing person with a bionic ear that could now be detached at will.

Replacement nose

Likewise a missing nose poses a great problem for replacement prosthesis, as in the past it had either to be glued on to the face or attached to a pair of spectacles. Both these methods were highly unsatisfactory as the glue could melt at an inopportune time or the spectacles become dislodged with nose attached. The rigid connection of a prosthetic nose to implants placed in the facial bone provides a realistic and reliable replacement.

Replacement eye

The loss of an eye can occur as a consequence of trauma or cancer surgery. This was the case for Bernie Cahill, a remarkable lady who underwent surgery to help control her cancer. She lost not only her eye but a considerable amount of bone and tissue around her eye socket, making it impossible for any kind of prosthesis to be retained. This cosmetic defect made it extremely difficult for this gregarious lady to enjoy a social life. Fig. 9.16 shows the extent of the defect, the implants in place and Bernie holding the eye prosthesis. Fig. 9.17 shows the prosthesis securely retained in place. Although the replacement eye cannot move in tandem with the good one, the results are extremely

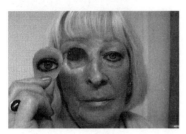

Fig. 9.16

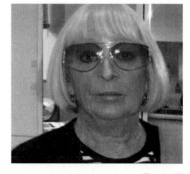

Fig. 9.17

realistic and give a very natural appearance. The reconstruction added greatly to Bernie's quality of life and her family have kindly given permission for her pictures and name to be used in this book as it might help other patients to know that this type of treatment is available in Ireland.

Facial and limb reconstructions

Major defects can sometimes arise from extensive surgery necessitated by the treatment of advanced cancer of the facial region. In extreme cases the nose, palate and cheekbone may be removed, leaving the patient in a difficult situation, as eating and speaking become virtually impossible. They may be so self-conscious that they cannot interact with other people and may end up leading a very restricted life indoors. Once again dental implants have been used to support extensive prosthesis that can replaces the palate, teeth, eye and facial tissues. Dr Osama Omar, consultant in maxillofacial prosthetics in the School of Dental Science, Trinity College Dublin, and Dr Eddie Cotter in private practice have been leading the way in Ireland in providing these types of prostheses. Extensive reconstructions have returned patients to a degree of normality, whereby they can eat, speak and interact successfully in society.

In the field of orthopaedic and hand surgery, Brånemark's team was able to replace missing thumbs and indeed whole limbs, using

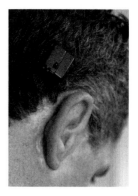

Fig. 9.18
© Cochlear™. Reproduced with permission.

prosthesis attached to titanium implants. Unlike other patients with prosthetic replacements that are not directly inserted into the remaining bone, these patients regain a sense of proprioception – a technical term to describe the ability to sense the touch and position of the prosthesis during function. This in turn allows for small and precise movements to be completed using the prosthesis.

Bone-Anchored Hearing Aids

One excellent application of implants is for patients who suffer from deafness as a result of conditions that prevent the conduction of sound waves to the inner ear. This is often a congenital condition, present from birth.

A corrective device was designed to attach to implants inserted into the temporal bone (a small bone in the skull just above the ear). This electronic device is known as a BAHA – Bone Anchored Hearing Aid. With BAHA the amplified signals are now directly transmitted into the inner ear via the direct connection through the temporal bone. Hearing is restored and, with training, these patients can enter a different world of hearing and ability to speak. Fig. 9.18 shows a patient with a bone-anchored hearing aid in place as well as a prosthetic ear. In this instance the treatment was not only cosmetic but helped to restore hearing. Such treatment is being made available by ENT surgeons in conjunction with audiologists in several specialist units in Ireland.

Dental Tourism:
It's All a Matter of Trust!

What is a cynic? A man who knows the price of everything
and the value of nothing.
Oscar Wilde (1854-1900), *Lady Windermere's Fan* (1892)

Price is what you pay. Value is what you get.
Warren Buffet (b. 1930)

The past ten years have seen a growing interest in a new kind of
tourism – dental and medical tourism. Many patients from Ireland
have travelled abroad to have extensive dental and medical treatment
carried out. The majority have gone to European countries but some
have sought help farther afield.

The most common reason for this new tourism is the perceived
high cost of treatment, especially in Ireland, when compared to low-
cost treatment offered elsewhere. At first, it was a word-of-mouth
process but once some overseas dental clinics became aware of the
potential market in Ireland, they started to place advertisements
in newspapers and magazines. They hoped that this would attract
many Irish people to take a cheap flight to other parts of Europe,
especially eastern European countries, and even as far afield as India
and Thailand. The trickle became a flood and the media became
interested, reinforcing the popular belief that high-quality dentistry
was available outside Ireland for half the price.

Low-cost dentistry is undoubtedly promoted in many overseas
locations. The clinics providing these services have gained enormously

from the considerable, if often uncritical, coverage of their activities on radio chat shows as well as in newspaper and magazine articles. Sometimes journalists, who have themselves travelled abroad for treatment, write these features. Happy patients are keen to tell their stories about the huge differential between the amounts quoted for treatment at home and what they paid abroad. These costs sometimes include travel, hotel accommodation and transport to the dental clinic as well as lifetime guarantees on all work carried out. It sounds wonderful, almost too good to be true. Sadly, in some cases, that's exactly what it has turned out to be.

Everyone has the right to seek better value healthcare and this includes dental treatment. However, as in many areas of life, lower costs do not always equate with better value. This elementary fact is sometimes lost in many of the pronouncements made by consumer bodies that often have no means at their disposal to evaluate the quality of service that healthcare patients receive. They measure price against price, ignoring the quality of treatment outcomes and the absolute necessity for regular follow-up, maintenance and aftercare. They usually pay only lip service to the possibility of short- or long-term clinical problems and complications arising and the potential difficulties, as well as cost, of undergoing any remedial treatment that might subsequently be required. In all fairness, they are probably blissfully unaware of the reality of these problems. They can only highlight the comparative prices for different 'items of treatment'. When applied to invasive surgical procedures and complex dental treatment, such an approach is full of pitfalls, as some Irish patients have found out to their cost.

In this chapter I will try to provide some clarity on these matters and discuss the significant difficulties and risks you may face when travelling abroad for treatment – especially if the treatment goes wrong, as this is mainly when real problems are encountered. In addition, I will provide some guidance on what you can do to protect yourself and the important role of the Irish Dental Council in helping you do so.

Cost/value and quality

There is an important assumption embedded in the 'lowest price method' of choosing which dental clinic to attend, as it requires an acceptance that the quality of what is on offer is much the same everywhere and that the only differential is price.

This is simply not true. Someone once said that there's an answer to every problem that's simple, obvious – and wrong. This is certainly the case with the lowest-price approach to dental treatment. Following this path can cause significant difficulties for a patient seeking not just low cost but good care and good value. The 'tourism' bit in the phrase 'dental tourism' provides a clue to understanding the underlying problem.

Let's take a look at tourism in general. When you book a holiday abroad you will know from the brochure or the website whether you have booked a five, four, three, or two star hotel or a bed and breakfast. The quality ratings are usually well controlled in individual countries and the relevant tourist bodies inspect the properties. If an agency sells a holiday that falls short of the brochure description you can go to court and seek compensation.

However, when you go abroad for healthcare, no such reliable grading system exists to provide you, in advance, with indications of the quality of the professionals into whose hands you are entrusting yourself. One of the most promoted areas of healthcare tourism is dental tourism. The fact is that there is often no objective, authoritative source that can reliably tell you anything about the professional standards of the people to whom you propose to entrust the care of your mouth.

Dentistry is not like a consumer product. It doesn't consist of manufactured items for purchase. If you want to buy a fridge or a flat-screen television you can research advertisements or catalogues for the best price. You can go anywhere and come back with the cheapest unit you can find. If it breaks down next year when the guarantee runs out, you throw it out and get another one without much heartbreak or very serious implications for your budget or your health. Not so with complex dental treatment and especially dental implants. If things go wrong, considerable amounts of treatment, including extensive surgery, may become necessary to rectify the situation. Apart from the pain and suffering that may arise from the complications, remedial treatment is always more expensive than the original treatment, takes considerably more time and, normally, cannot easily replicate the results that might have been obtained had the treatment been successful in the first place. Should this happen to a patient who has had low-cost treatment carried out abroad, the original treatment may prove to have been an expensive exercise.

Quality of care

I am not claiming that you cannot receive high-quality dental care anywhere other than the Republic of Ireland or that nothing can go wrong if treatment is provided in this country. To make such assertions would be ridiculous as well as untrue. Dentists in Ireland may be proud of what we do and how we do it but of course we acknowledge that, in all developed countries, dentists, surgeons, technicians and support staff are to be found who are perfectly well trained to provide a high standard of care.

The difficulty facing the dental tourist is in finding the right clinic. To be fair, it should also be said that having the treatment in Ireland cannot provide you with a cast-iron guarantee that you will always receive the very best of care. However, at least, you can undergo treatment here with the reassuring knowledge that there are considerable safeguards in place to look after your best interests.

I have lectured in a number of the tourist destination countries and can testify that there are usually many excellent undergraduate and specialist-training dentistry programmes in place, as well as high academic standards. However, some of my colleagues in these countries are less than enamoured of the activities of a few of the clinics that advertise abroad to promote dental tourism. When I meet colleagues from all over the world one thing becomes abundantly clear: good dentists in every country are already in demand and busy providing care to their own population and have little need to import patients from abroad.

Potential pitfalls

Caveat emptor (let the buyer beware)

Despite these issues, if you decide to take the consumer approach of seeking the lowest-cost care by travelling overseas, you should at least adopt a basic tenet of consumer awareness, summed up in the phrase *caveat emptor* – 'Let the buyer beware.' Remember that if, right now, you are unhappy enough with your teeth, or lack of them, to consider taking a flight to an overseas country to have major treatment, you really need to protect yourself from ending up in an even worse situation. If you wish to avoid this, do some research before you entrust the care of your precious mouth to an unknown clinic.

Patients who are unfortunate enough to have developed problems after receiving implant treatment abroad are frequently referred to a specialist in Ireland, either in private practice or in one of the dental schools. Clearly, I am not referring to patients who have had satisfactory treatment carried out but to those for whom the treatment has gone wrong – usually very wrong. In these circumstances we will do everything possible to help remedy the situation. It is of no consolation to the individual patient to know that their case might represent only a percentage of those who undertake dental tourism. The misery they feel about their own disastrous results can well edge into fury when they consider not just the original price but the extensive treatment often necessary to repair any damage and the total cost of this treatment.

What is worrying is that the numbers of patients presenting with problems appears to be increasing. This may be because higher numbers are travelling. However, it is also a reality that it can take a few years after the treatment has been completed for underlying problems to make their appearance. The most common problem reported in an Irish Dental Association survey of treatment abroad was that unnecessary dental work was carried out. This is known as 'overprescribing' and can lead to many perfectly good teeth being crowned or root-canal treated, albeit at 'low cost'. Should a tooth that requires no treatment be attacked in this way, not only has the patient been duped into paying money for treatment that was not required in the first place but, far worse, this can set the scene for future problems. It is worth remembering that a natural, healthy untreated tooth is the gold standard for longevity and health. Crowns, veneers and root treatments all have their place in treating diseased and unsightly teeth but, when they are used on healthy teeth without any good reason and especially if inexpertly carried out, the results will always be to the patient's disadvantage. Overprescribing is a gross breach of the ethics and integrity that underlie the profession of dentistry. In the unlikely event that a dentist fully registered with the Irish Dental Council were found guilty of this he/she would almost certainly have their names erased from the Dental Register and be unable to continue to practice in the Republic of Ireland.

One extreme example of dental tourism going badly wrong concerns several patients who had all been treated in one particular overseas clinic. Responding to a newspaper advertisement offering low-cost dental implants they attended for a consultation in a hotel room in south Dublin. With the patient seated in a hotel chair a dentist was apparently able to work out the requirements and procedures for complex treatments. Undeterred by the torchlight examination, many of the prospective patients signed up and travelled abroad. They underwent extensive and complex treatment in a pleasantly appointed clinic. Some of the treatment plans included implants and some of the implants required additional bone-grafting procedures.

Apart from serious questions about the level of infection control that can be provided in these circumstances, it would be an understatement to say that a superficial examination, such as has been described, is not acceptable best practice. It should have been a clear warning about the quality of care that was likely to result. Complex implant treatments always require a thorough evaluation of the patient with appropriate x-rays and, sometimes, special CT scans. The final result needs to be visualised in advance and usually transferred to study plaster casts so that the surgeon can see exactly where to place the implants. The opinion of more than one dentist or specialist may be necessary to ensure an optimum result for the treatment, especially when there are complex problems to be addressed.

Such a careful and detailed analysis, carried out within the context of a patient's overall dental and medical health status, gives the best chance of obtaining a predictable long-term result. It also allows dentists to inform patients fully about the procedures they are about to undergo and guide their expectations as to the final result that can reasonably be expected. Such an approach provides a basis for an informed discussion with the patient about the benefits, drawbacks and possible complications of the proposed treatment, as compared to alternative methods. As a patient it is important that you are never rushed into accepting complex treatments. Time should be allowed for you to consider the treatment proposal and you should be provided with an opportunity for further discussion about any aspect of your proposed care you are not clear about. This time delay is an essential component in ensuring that you are fully informed about the treatment to which you are consenting.

The problem was that no Irish dentist was aware of these torchlight examinations until long after they happened. The first most of us learned of it was when patients turned up in our clinics, in pain, in distress and, in some cases, suffering from severe infections. For the individual patients concerned it was an unmitigated dental disaster.

It might sound as if I am condemning all overseas clinics on the basis of the behaviour of one establishment. This is not the case. My real purpose is to draw attention to how difficult it can be for a lay prospective patient to make any realistic judgement about the quality of care they are likely to receive.

All a matter of trust

When you choose to undergo treatment with a dentist it is a trans-action very much based on trust. Patients are rarely in a position to verify in advance the necessity of the treatment recommended or the efficacy of the treatment to be provided. This leaves them in a very vulnerable position. Should they decide to proceed with treatment it means they trust the dentist and assume that he/she will always act in their best interests, as they are ethically obliged to do. Dr Eleanor O'Higgins, a faculty member of the UCD School of Business, writes about the essential role of trust in the relationship between patients and dentists in an article in the *Journal of the Irish Dental Association* (August 2014). In her article Dr O'Higgins identifies three criteria that we use to judge someone as trustworthy in this context: competency, benevolence and integrity. All three must be present in order for us to trust someone. In Ireland if someone is fully registered with the Dental Council competency is assumed. Benevolence represents a belief that the professional involved will always have the interests of the patient at heart, while integrity arises from the perception that the dentist abides by a set of principles that is consistent with the values and needs of the patient. Traditionally, benevolence and integrity were mostly built up by long-term relationships with a patient's general dental practitioner and word-of-mouth recommendations from existing patients. Specialists depended on their reputation within the dental community to ensure that patients would be referred to them.

Common fallacies

It is worth highlighting some common fallacies that can lead you astray in relation to judging the quality of care you might receive:

1. *Full-page advertisements and professionally crafted websites will provide reliable information about the quality of care and treatment provided by a practice.*

Thus is not necessarily true because all these marketing tools can simply be purchased to convey a veneer of professionalism. No particular dental skills are required to obtain them. If you decide, 'These people wouldn't be in business and have the lovely premises in the photographs if they weren't reputable,' you may be one step on the path to disaster. The same principle applies to people who choose to buy prescription drugs from online pharmacies on impressive websites only to find that they have purchased dud medications. Additionally, website patient testimonials can be selective, unverifiable and unreliable and, as a result, deeply misleading.

In the Republic of Ireland the Irish Dental Council is charged with regulating the content of advertisements and websites produced for dentists. From time to time they circulate guidelines to all dentists on the dental register regarding acceptable, truthful and ethical practice in this area. They also reserve the right to inspect any testimonials posted to verify that they are genuine. They have no jurisdiction whatsoever over websites or advertisements that promote treatment for Irish patients outside the country. The Dental Council is active in this area and does takes action but it would need huge resources to police and investigate everything that is posted. In her article Dr O'Higgins expresses this opinion:

> Of course, nowadays, the internet and social media allow for speedy word of mouth reporting of experiences with particular professionals. Isn't there a website called, 'Rate my dentist'? Of course such websites are not always influenced by high-minded moral principles and are unfortunately open to abuse, so we have to be careful about trusting those websites themselves!

Websites do have an important role. They can give you a good sense of the type, location and opening times of the practices that are being promoted, the range and cost of services being offered and information on the profiles and activities of the professionals and staff who will be involved with your care.

2. *All dentists in Europe receive more or less the same undergraduate training, sit similar exams and therefore have much the same competencies on graduation.*

This may be true but it misses the point. No undergraduate education can prepare anyone for a lifetime in practice in a field that is constantly changing. A sound basic training can prepare dentists to enter a lifetime commitment to continuing professional development and it is this process that will determine the quality of care that they deliver. This is true whether one decides to become involved in general dental practice or continues in postgraduate education to specialist level.

Newly qualified graduates in many countries may start out with much the same level of qualification but, ten years later, there can be a significant divergence in the quality of care they are able to offer. Some websites and brochures list a number of courses the dentist has attended. It is extremely difficult for members of the public to evaluate whether or not these have any real value. At one extreme, some courses listed may have important-sounding names but can turn out to be little more than a seminar provided by a dental company or manufacturer that took place in a hotel room over a period of one or two days. Courses of this kind are sometimes listed by dentists who may have undergone little or no formal postgraduate training to give the impression that they are better qualified than they are. Sometimes courses are not even mentioned but vague references are given, such as 'travelling to America to keep abreast of the latest developments'.

This is not always the case. Sometimes overseas dentists, in common with many Irish dentists, gain further qualification and expertise by attending courses that require a commitment by the practitioner of a year or more and provide extensive training in the subject. This indicates good continuing professional development.

Undergraduate dental education in Ireland is of the highest standard and postgraduate dental programmes ensure a very high level of specialist training. Because of this, dentists trained in Ireland have always enjoyed easy access to postgraduate training in North

America and Europe. An example of this is that, in 2012, the Commission on Dental Accreditation of Canada (CDAC) reached a reciprocal agreement with the Irish Dental Council to recognise the qualifications of dentists trained in Ireland, a recognition that allows them to practise in Canada. Irish dentists are also very enthusiastic participants in continuing professional development activities. There is an extensive annual programme of postgraduate courses and scientific symposia for general dental practitioners provided under the auspices of the Irish Dental Association, the university teaching hospitals and the Royal College of Surgeons in Ireland, as well as some specialist organisations. General practitioners can also obtain postgraduate qualifications by engaging in part-time courses. The practitioner enrolment in these activities is high and contributes significantly to awareness of new developments in dental practice and to high standards of care. As a specialist I see many patients referred for treatment by general practitioner colleagues in Ireland and I can testify to the high standard of their work and professionalism in the treatment of the vast majority of these patients.

3. *Memberships of associations and what may appear to be learned societies are important.*

Once again these can be very misleading. An example of this is 'Fellow of the Royal Society of Medicine in London'. It sounds impressive. Very impressive. However the only requirements for election are two nominations and a membership fee. Although it is a learned institution that encourages and carries out important research in the medical and dental fields, it does not provide any formal training in dentistry. Nor does it set any examinations. Nor does it issue diplomas. So to be a Fellow of the Royal Society of Medicine may be worthwhile (I certainly find it so) but it carries no implication whatsoever of higher levels of qualification or expertise. Many other associations and societies have similar prerequisites for membership. Whilst most well-qualified practitioners will be members of established organisations catering for their specific interests, membership alone does not necessarily equate with advanced training or expertise. It is really confusing for a member of the public to know what to make of this.

The Irish Dental Council does not recognise such memberships as evidence of qualifications or training. The only additional qualifications that can be registered on the lists of duly qualified dentists and specialists maintained by the Dental Council are those awarded by approved dental education authorities. All this information is available to the general public.

4.   *If someone is a dental implant specialist they must be good.*

Well, they might be, were it not for one minor problem: in Ireland there is no such thing as a dental implant specialist. Nor, in the view of many of us, should there be. Orthopaedic and plastic surgeons place many different types of implants and it would never occur to them to describe themselves as 'implant specialists'. The dental implant in itself, although important, does not constitute a total treatment and its role is to support replacements for missing teeth. In fact the successful practice of the full range of dental implant treatment requires a broad spectrum of skills in both surgery and prosthodontics. Some general dental practitioners who have undergone further training also provide implant treatment as part of general dental activities.

The EU currently recognises only two dental specialisms: oral surgery and orthodontics. This is the official position in Ireland. Members with qualifications in these two specialisms are registered with the Dental Council, which will provide a list if requested. However, many other individual countries recognise a further number of specialisms, for example periodontics (gum disorders). In the context of implants periodontists are fully trained in the surgical placement of implants and associated procedures. Other specialisms include endodontics (root canal treatments), prosthodontics (crowns, bridgework, dentures), paedodontics (dental services for children) and special needs dentistry. In the Republic of Ireland we have many graduates who have undergone full-time formal training of at least three years in these specialisms either abroad or in the dental schools in Dublin and Cork. The Department of Health and Children is long overdue in providing its approval to allow these well-trained specialists to be officially recognised and registered and it is clearly in the interest of the general public that this should happen. In the meantime they are providing an excellent service to the community, even if the public cannot easily identify who they are except by means of the recommendation of another dentist.

Information about health regulators and professional bodies in other countries can be obtained on these websites: www. healthregulations.org and www.fedcar.eu.

What happens if things go wrong?

Many overseas clinics offer a guarantee that, if complications develop as a result of the treatment provided, remedial care will be provided at no additional charge.

This sounds great – but what actually happens when things go seriously wrong? Taking advantage of this guarantee often proves to be impracticable for the patient who has had complex implant treatments that subsequently develop complications. In my experience this is a major danger in having such treatment carried out abroad. Although no further professional fees may be levied by the clinic, the cost of travelling, perhaps numerous times, as well as the time involved, must be taken into account. It is often the case that remedial treatment cannot be completed in short visits and a lack of progress or worsening of the problems can eventually lead to the patient giving up on the whole process and seeking corrective treatment at home. In my experience some of these overseas clinics may not even be around at a future date to honour the guarantees they promote.

The Irish Dental Council advice is very clear on the subject of aftercare:

'You should ensure that you are satisfied with arrangements for follow-up care should there be complications. This facility may not be in place or may be difficult to access.

'You should be satisfied as to how financial matters will be resolved if costs escalate, such as in the case of complications, as legal recourse may be limited or difficult to obtain.'

Unfortunately, it may only be at this point, when things have gone seriously wrong, that the patient will become aware that it may prove impossible for them to get any redress for their failed treatment, even if a poor standard of care or negligence was involved. Why is this so?

In theory it should be possible to seek redress through the legal system in the country where the treatment is carried out. Patients soon discover, however, that many formidable practical difficulties will need to be overcome.

Firstly, there is the cost involved in identifying and engaging a lawyer who deals in medical negligence in another country. All proceedings will take place in the language of that country, expert witnesses willing to give evidence on behalf of the patient will need to be found and paid for and a court or tribunal appearance may well be necessary.

Negligence laws, procedures and awards also vary from country to country and there can be no guarantee that the court will find in favour of the patient and award costs. The reality is that very few, if any claims are successfully pursued in this way.

A further difficulty may be the extent and scope of the professional indemnity insurance (if any) held by the dentist involved.

Safeguards available in Ireland
The Irish Dental Council

In Ireland there are many safeguards in place to protect the patient. The most important is the Irish Dental Council, the statutory body that regulates all aspects of the practice of dentistry, including overseeing the outcomes of undergraduate and postgraduate dental education in Ireland.

It is important to emphasise that the Dental Council is not there to protect dentists: its unequivocal duty is to protect the interests of the public in their professional relationship with dentists. Although the Council includes dentists, some elected by their peers and some appointed by the universities, it also includes members who are not dentists. Among the many duties of the Council is the maintenance of a list of all dentists legally allowed to practise within the state, including details of their qualifications. The Council also maintains a list of registered dental specialists and has a fitness-to-practice committee that will investigate complaints from the general public about alleged professional misconduct and unfitness to practise.

If the committee decides there is a case to be answered the dentist in question will be called to a special hearing. If a dentist is found to have fallen seriously below the standard of care or professional behaviour that might reasonably be expected they can be subject to disciplinary sanctions, including, in the most serious cases, suspension or erasure of registration. Erasure of their name from the dental register prevents that person from practising dentistry in Ireland.

The scope of activity of the Council is strictly limited to those whose name appears on the Dental Register for the Republic of Ireland. It has no jurisdiction whatsoever elsewhere; nor can it deal directly with complaints about dentists outside the Republic of Ireland. Most countries will have a regulatory body of some sort, usually referred to as 'the competent authority'. However, language and other procedural difficulties can make it virtually impossible for an Irish patient to pursue an overseas dentist based in a different country through the local regulatory body.

The Irish Dental Association

A new Dental Complaints Resolution Service was recently introduced in Ireland. This independent service has the backing of the Irish Dental Association and will provide an opportunity for patients who have complaints about, or who are in dispute with their dentist, to have their problems sorted out in a fair and timely manner with the help of an experienced mediator. The service is intended to deal with most complaints about dental care and treatment in the Republic of Ireland, covering such areas as treatment standards, diagnosis, communications, professional etiquette and fees.

This service is free of charge and may enable patients to avoid the costly process of initiating legal proceedings. If the patient remains dissatisfied with the outcome they will not have prejudiced their rights to request a hearing with the Dental Council of Ireland or to initiate legal proceedings. The Irish legal system provides for a patient to sue a dentist for negligence and, if successful, for financial compensation to be awarded for any remedial treatment, damages or any loss suffered.

Professional indemnity

In Ireland most Irish-trained dentists and doctors belong to a medical or dental indemnity agency or insurance company. The largest of these is Dental Protection Ltd, which provides unlimited indemnity for dentists against claims of negligence. The company also runs educational and risk management programmes to help dentists avoid making errors and to ensure that they are fully aware of their responsibilities to patients. Members are also covered for any claims made for treatment that was carried out while they were members, even if the claim arises much later and they are no longer members. If it is clear that a mistake was made, or treatment falls below an accepted standard of care, then, in most cases, a settlement is likely be reached, without the need to go to court. Apart from providing peace of mind for dentists, the system provides a fund for patients who successfully pursue a claim.

It is my view that appropriate indemnity or insurance represents an essential safeguard for patients. At present, although the Irish Dental Council states that it is an ethical requirement to have such insurance, it is not mandatory. I am of the opinion that it should become a statutory requirement for practising dentists in this country. This would require a change to the Dental Act that governs the practice of dentistry in Ireland and is in the process of being reviewed. I hope it will be one of the areas to be addressed.

Are there any steps I can take to protect myself?

The Irish Dental Council website provides advice under the heading 'Having Treatment Abroad'. This includes eleven questions that prospective patients should consider before undertaking any such treatment. The Council suggests that the following questions should be read in conjunction with the advice provided in their publication, *Choosing Your Dentist*:

1. How will I determine the qualifications and experience of the dentist who will be treating me when I am abroad? (If a dentist claims to be a specialist it is important to ask whether they can support this claim. Some European countries hold registers of dentists entitled to use the title 'specialist'.)
2. Will the dental team who will be treating me be able to communicate with me in a language I will understand?
3. What aftercare will be provided?
4. If I need any remedial work and have to return to the country where the procedures were carried out, who pays for flights, accommodation and the additional work needed?
5. Does the dentist have adequate professional indemnity cover to carry out all dental/surgical treatment, including specialised procedures?
6. What are my legal rights if something goes wrong with the treatment that is provided or if I am unhappy with the result?
7. If I need remedial work for any reason including pain, bleeding or infection and do not want to travel back to the country where the original treatment was carried out, can I have it done at home?
8. How will this be organised for me? Who will pay?
9. Who can I contact for advice after treatment?
10. Will my records be kept in my language or the local language?
11. Will I be given all my records after treatment?

If you have received implant treatment, records take on a special importance, because maintenance or remedial work is likely to be required at a future date. These days, there are very many different implant systems on the market. Most have their own components that are not interchangeable with others. Some are cheaper copycats or clones of more established products. It is important that replacement components that are compatible with your implants be available in ten or even twenty years' time. The major implant companies have an excellent record in this regard but some of the clone manufacturers may not. It is very distressing when a patient develops problems and finds that no components are available to match the implant system that was used for their treatment. Patients are advised to ask for details of all components used for implant treatment. Where possible, copies of the stickers that accompany the components should be provided, showing the name of the manufacturer of the implant and attached components, as well as individual batch numbers.

It might never occur to most patients undergoing implant surgery in Ireland to ask for such documentation, although nowadays they should ensure it is available. However, when a patient is undergoing surgery of this kind overseas, it is absolutely imperative that they receive every last detail in order to ensure that their implants can be maintained in Ireland or elsewhere for decades to come.

Nor is it just a matter of retaining paperwork: you should also keep any models or records on which the crown or bridgework that attach to the implants are based. If subsequent remedial work is required and is not being provided by the original clinic, these records will be invaluable and may help to reduce costs.

Many people do not consider going to Northern Ireland for dental treatment as dental tourism. It's easy to head north of the border and there's absolutely no reason to reject the idea of such a trip but, as always, do choose carefully. It will come as no surprise that Northern Ireland has a lower cost base than the Republic, which allows dentists working there to charge less. This is also why dentistry in practices in the west end of London can be considerably dearer than in Belfast or, indeed, Dublin. I collaborate with many colleagues from the north of Ireland and the Dental School in Queen's University Belfast provides excellent training.

As always, in my opinion, the best way to choose a practice is on the recommendation of people or dentists who live locally and who will be aware of the dental practices that have well-deserved reputations. In fact the same principle applies when it comes to choosing a dentist anywhere in the world. Be especially careful if you are led to believe that complex dental treatments, involving multiple crowns and bridgework, will be completed in a matter of days if a general dentist or specialist in Ireland has advised you that it will take much longer to provide this treatment. In my opinion, if practices use paid agents to recruit patients, it is a sure sign that they are engaged in dentistry as a business, rather than committed to it as an important component of overall healthcare. Don't forget that it is always a matter of whom you are going to trust.

With regard to costs, the post-Celtic Tiger economic situation in Ireland has also affected dentists. As a result treatment costs have significantly decreased here and dentists have introduced greater efficiencies in the delivery of care. Dentistry is highly competitive in Ireland, especially when the patient factors in the standard of treatment delivered and the availability of essential and knowledgeable local follow-up care and responsibility.

Eyes wide shut

In summary, by all means consider combining a holiday with dental treatment overseas but do not let the holiday aspect cloud your judgement, as there are many important considerations to take into account. Before rushing to sign up for low-cost dental tourism and grab yourself a bargain, at the very least read the advice provided the Irish Dental Council. In 2010 they published guidelines for patients, 'Choosing your Dentist' and 'Going Abroad for Dental Treatment'. (Some excerpts from these appear in this chapter.) These authoritative publications are a must-read for anyone who needs independent, unbiased advice from the statutory regulatory body in Ireland and they can be accessed on the council's website: www.dentalcouncil.ie.

Friendly receptionists and a warm and welcoming greeting from office staff, who may go to the trouble of picking you up at the airport or railway station, can certainly make for a very pleasant experience, but, in fact, tell you little or nothing about the competence of the dentists who will provide your care. No matter where you seek treatment, whether at home or abroad, do not make a choice based solely on media advertising, websites or promotional literature. If possible always seek confirmation advice from general dental practitioners or specialists. Make sure you read and follow the Dental Council guidelines and don't make the lowest cost your only criterion. Remember: if you seek out only the cheapest, that's what you will get!

Frequently Asked Questions

What are dental implants?

Modern dental implants are inserts that are surgically placed within the jawbone, where they function in a similar way to the root of a tooth. The vast majority are shaped like screws and are made of titanium. Those with the longest track record of success are made from commercially pure titanium. When teeth have been lost, dental implants are used to provide support for tooth replacements such as crowns, bridges and dentures. The tooth replacements that attach to the implants are known as prostheses.

Are dental implant treatments successful?

This is an important question as it concerns much more than simply how long dental implants can be expected to last. The yardstick for success for an individual patient will be how close the completed treatment comes to fulfilling their expectations. This is why there is so much emphasis throughout this book on the necessity of gaining a thorough understanding of each patient's problems and expectations. Each patient is unique. In addition, expectations can be very high and sometimes unattainable, especially if they are gleaned from website pictures showing beautiful results and giving glowing short-term testimonials.

The reality is that patients will judge treatment success in terms of how well it improves their function, comfort and appearance and to what extent the final result helps overcome any disability (physical, psychological or emotional) they have experienced as a result of losing teeth or from wearing dentures. The planning of treatment should always begin with a comprehensive examination and a visualisation of the proposed result: only then can the optimum surgical placement of implants be planned. This alone can take several visits.

How long will dental implants last?
This will depend on four factors:

1. The training, skill and experience of the team providing the treatment
2. The suitability of the patient for the procedures undertaken
3. The commitment of the patient to maintaining good oral hygiene and attending for routine professional cleaning and monitoring
4. The type of implant used

Implants placed in the lower jaw in patients with no natural teeth can potentially last a lifetime. An overall success rate of 98 per cent has been recorded with them over twenty years, a figure that coincides with my own experience over thirty years. Implants placed in the upper jaw are less successful, with a rate as low as 92-96 per cent. Overall, however, when conditions are right and the treatment is carried out to a high standard, implants can provide the best long-term outcomes when compared to conventional bridgework, crowns or dentures.

In some cases, bone loss can occur around implants and lead to localised infections (perimplantitis) which, if left untreated, can eventually result in failure. Patients have an important role to play in how long implants will last: they must maintain meticulous oral hygiene procedures and attend for visits with a dental hygienist or dentist at regular intervals so that any deterioration can be detected early and treated.

How long does treatment take?
This can vary from a matter of hours to many months. Irrespective of how long the treatment takes, all patients must undergo a thorough clinical examination, supplemented by x-rays. Additional

investigations such as a study cast, diagnostic wax-up or CT scan may also be needed. Time is required to understand exactly what the patient wants from the treatment and to establish what their main priorities are. Only in this way can a treatment plan be drawn up that addresses a patient's individual problems, needs and expectations. This plan must include the possibility of alternative treatments and, most importantly, take into consideration any limitations as to what can be achieved. In my experience, this will take a minimum of two visits and, with complex cases, a lot longer. If one short, cursory examination with a single x-ray is all that is carried out prior to treatment, patients should take this as a warning sign and perhaps consider obtaining a second opinion. Above all, never allow yourself to be rushed into a decision.

If additional procedures such as bone or gum grafts need to be undertaken, this will add to the time taken for completion. Great care and patience are required to ensure the best functional and aesthetic results.

What are Teeth in a Day?

This widely-used term describes the process of undergoing implant surgery and having the replacement teeth fitted on the same day, an alternative to the more traditional technique of allowing the implants to undergo a period of healing before making and fitting the prosthesis. It does not necessarily apply to any special technique and some techniques of this kind may not have any documentation to prove long-term success.

At Blackrock Clinic (www.blackrockclinicdental.ie) we began to offer Same Day Teeth in 1999. The procedure was filmed by Channel 4 and subsequently broadcast on *The Richard and Judy Show*. Since then the process has become technically more sophisticated, with computerised planning and Cad/Cam production of the prosthesis. In addition, simplified techniques have been developed that allow for successful outcomes at lower cost.

Using as little as four implants, a full upper or lower denture can be replaced by an implant-supported prosthesis (not removable by the patient).

It should be noted that although this treatment is carried out in one day the same requirements for thorough examination and planning will apply and these will normally take several visits.

It is our experience that not every patient is suitable for this treatment. From our long experience we have also found that the surgery and prosthodontic skills required to produce a successful result are of a very high order. These, in my opinion, are best provided by an experienced specialist-trained team.

Will I be able to eat all kinds of food and live a normal life after I have had implant treatment?

If you have been wearing conventional removable dentures and, as a result, you have found that your diet has become restricted or that you have suffered badly from loss of appearance, confidence and self-esteem, implants-supported prosthesis can transform your life. Let me remind you of what M.W., a forty-two-year-old female patient, who had all her upper and lower teeth restored by means of dental implants, said (Chapter 8):

> I would like to take this opportunity to thank you for changing my life and giving me back my confidence…I had lost all my confidence and hated the fact that I had lost so many teeth and had to wear dentures. It's very difficult to explain to anyone how that feels. I couldn't eat properly and would avoid going to restaurants with friends. I even tried not to laugh or smile so that I wouldn't show my teeth. This is not the way to live your life…
>
> My life has really changed for the better and I am always smiling now. It's amazing how free I feel and how I don't avoid photos or eating out.
>
> Apart from the cosmetic side of things I no longer have pain or difficulty in eating certain foods. I love eating fruit and nuts and I don't even have to think about whether I can or not now. In fact I

think my implants are even stronger than my own teeth.

I would highly recommend implants to any one who has dentures and not to wait for years to have them done.

My brother made a calendar for my mother for Christmas and put a photo of each family member on the date of their birthday and any other special occasion. He called me to see if I had any photos of me smiling as he had lots but I wasn't smiling in any of his. Guess what – neither did I!!! I can't wait for this year's calendar!

Will the teeth on my implants look like natural teeth?

When the missing teeth are in what is known as the 'aesthetic zone', this can represent a significant challenge. The aesthetic zone lies towards the front of the mouth and if a patient shows the gum tissues above the teeth when they smile (a high smile line), particular care is necessary. When such a patient loses a tooth there will be changes to the gum tissues and underlying bone and this is exactly the place from which a replacement implant-supported tooth will emerge. Sometimes a localised bone or gum tissue graft will be required to compensate for these changes, something that should be discussed in advance. In other situations the patient's lips will reveal only the teeth attached to the implants and not the gum tissues. All individuals are different and the likely results need to be discussed and visualised. Generally the overall improvement in appearance is excellent but in particularly difficult cases a team approach involving a prosthodontist and a surgeon will achieve the best outcome.

If I have been wearing dentures for a long time will placing implants be more problematic?

Generally this is more of a problem with upper teeth replacements than lower ones, something I have discussed in detail in Chapter 8. It is very rare that nothing can be done but some treatment may involve additional surgical and prosthodontic procedures.

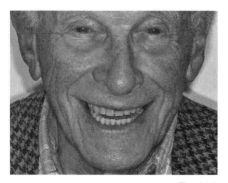
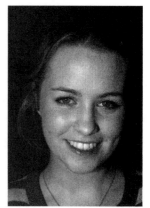

Fig. 11.1   Fig. 11.2

© Professor David Harris: reproduced with patients' permission.

Am I too old to have implant treatment?

Providing there are no medical contraindications to the procedure there does not appear to be any upper age limit for successful implant treatment, as bone will accept implants at any age. Fig. 11.1 shows the oldest patient I have ever treated who was aged eighty-nine at the time. He is now ninety-five years of age, having gone on to become the oldest student ever in Trinity College, Dublin.

Can I be too young for implants?

Yes. Implants in children and growing adolescents are contra-indicated and are best delayed until growth has stabilised. This can be a minimum of eighteen years of age for girls and twenty for boys. However when it is anticipated that implants will be required, much can be done in earlier years to ensure that implants will be successful. For example when teeth are lost or are congenitally absent, steps should be taken to maintain the space and bone for implants. The only exception to this rule is if the implants are being used to help teeth move as part of orthodontic treatment, not to replace teeth. Fig. 11.2 shows the youngest patient we have treated, aged eighteen.

I had a bad car accident and suffered serious damage to my mouth and jaw area, as well as losing all my front teeth. Would I be a suitable candidate for implants?

Implants and the teeth they support can play a significant role in restoring a patient to a more normal function and appearance following severe trauma of any kind – especially younger patients who can suffer badly from the sudden change to their body image. In the case of severe accidents the implants are usually considered after initial healing and necessary reconstructive surgery have been completed. Further surgery by a specialist oral surgeon may then be required, including bone and soft-tissue grafts, to make the damaged tissues suitable for implant placement. Because of these preliminary procedures treatments can take much longer than normal to complete.

Do I need to be admitted into hospital to have dental implants?

No, the vast majority of procedures can be carried out on outpatients under local anaesthesia or with supplemental intravenous sedation. Where extensive surgery is required, as with zygomatic implants or major bone grafting, general anaesthesia and an overnight stay in hospital may be necessary.

Is having dental implants placed painful?

The good news is that implant surgery is a very gentle procedure that, in my experience, is associated with little postoperative pain. Any discomfort can normally be well controlled by prescribed pain medication. As with any surgery there is always a chance of more severe pain in the postoperative period. Sometimes there is a reason for this, such as swelling, which may make the stitches tighten and become painful. In many practices, including my own, patients are supplied with out-of-hours telephone numbers and cover is provided at weekends to ensure that, in the unlikely event of serious problems, help is always at hand. My experience is that I am called on no more than about twice a year.

I am very nervous about dental treatment and I would prefer not to be aware during any surgery. Is there any way of helping me?

Although the thought of having dental implants placed can be very frightening, implant treatment is in fact a very gentle procedure. However, many patients prefer not to be aware during surgery, especially when multiple implants are to be placed. Should you wish it, treatment can be carried out using intravenous sedation to supplement the normal dental local anaesthesia (injection in the gum). An anaesthetist or a specially trained dentist administers the sedation prior to the local anaesthesia. This will ensure that the whole experience is made much more pleasant for you. You will feel very calm and have little if any memory of the entire surgery, including receiving the local anaesthesia. Over the past thirty years I have found that even our most nervous patients are entirely happy when they undergo treatment in this way. In situations when a full general anaesthetic is required this should be administered by a consultant anaesthetist within a hospital setting.

What complications can occur with implants?

Infections and bone loss as a result of infections can occur around dental implants and are often related to poor oral hygiene. Patients should attend for professional cleaning by a dentist or dental hygienist on a regular basis and carry out their own oral hygiene routine every day. A source of misunderstanding can be the fact that although the implants can last a patient's lifetime this is unlikely to be true for the teeth that attach to them. Breakages or wear and tear will occur, especially with overdentures and in people who grind or clench their teeth. This means that repairs or servicing will be required and some-times replacement prosthesis needed. As with all surgery there are uncommon or remote risks, including damage to adjacent anatomical features such as nerves, sinuses and natural teeth. Should general anaesthesia be required this has its own separate risks. Patients with any pertinent underlying disease should be carefully assessed to ensure that a particular treatment does not pose any special risk for them.

Every patient is different and surgery can vary in its extent. It is up to the surgeon involved to inform the patient of any particular risks that apply to them as part of the process of their consenting to treatment.

Could I be allergic to titanium?

The dental implants with the longest clinical trials and success rates are made from commercially pure titanium. The level of true allergy to this material is difficult to quantify but it is certainly very rare indeed, given its wide use in surgery and in the many millions of dental implants that have been placed. Some implants are made from a titanium alloy and theoretically it is possible to develop an allergy to any of the metals used in the alloy. If there is any possibility that you might be allergic to titanium you can be checked out by a medical specialist in the field of allergies. Do not rely on information from non-medically qualified practitioners or website information. Other types of implants can be used that do not contain titanium and are entirely free of metal but the long-term performance of these implants has yet to be established.

Are implants guaranteed?

Implants are highly successful when placed correctly in suitable situations and properly maintained by the patient and dentist. However, as with all surgical interventions, it would be unethical to give any absolute guarantee of success. All that can be guaranteed is that the best advice will be given and the surgeon and prosthodontist will use all their skill and experience to help achieve a successful outcome. It is not uncommon to see advertisements giving guarantees for life and claiming 'permanent' teeth replacements. Be aware that nothing is permanent in the mouth – not even natural teeth – and that some of the clinics offering lifetime guarantees may not be around to fulfil them (see Chapter 10).

Many practices, including our own, provide both a comprehensive and limited guarantee for a period of time, providing that the patient is a non-smoker and follows the maintenance protocols that are prescribed for them. Occasionally, there are special circumstances that might apply that would limit the guarantee: these should always be clearly understood and agreed in advance. In all situations, should problems arise outside the guarantee, we will try to solve them at the lowest outlay for the patient.

How much does implant treatment cost?

There are two main costs involved: firstly, the fee for the surgery to be carried out and the cost of the special implants and prosthetic components or materials used; and, secondly, the cost of making the prosthesis or teeth that are attached to the implants and attendance with a dental hygienist as required pre- and post- treatment. In addition, the costs of any special investigations such as study models, x-rays and CT scans, as well as diagnostic wax-ups specially ordered to visualise the end result, may be applicable. Patients should make sure that the fees quoted to them cover all these elements. Procedures such as bone or soft-tissue grafting as well as the type of prosthesis made will have an impact on the total costs. In general a fixed prosthesis that is not removable by the patient will cost more than an overdenture that attaches to the implants and is removed by the patient for cleaning. In all cases patients should receive a comprehensive cost breakdown before beginning treatment.

Will my health insurance provider cover implants?

This varies from one company to the next. Companies also apply various restrictions and limitations. For example, VHI has always provided cover for implants in the lower jaw when all the teeth have been lost. They will pay a fee toward the surgery and, most importantly, refund directly to the patient the cost of the implant components used – a sum that is significantly higher than the contribution to the surgical fee. Other healthcare providers pay only the lower contribution of the surgical fee, not the purchase cost of the components. Because there are frequent changes in different plan options the practitioner should apply to the insurance company involved on behalf of the patient and seek prior approval for implant treatment.

Is tax relief available for dental implant treatment?
Yes, at the time of publication both the implant surgery and any fixed prosthesis should be allowable against income tax in Ireland at the rate of 20 per cent under the terms and conditions of the Med 2 form. As the allowance is at the discretion of the Revenue Commissioners, patients should seek independent advice about how the relief might benefit them. The role of the dentist and surgeons involved is limited to providing the necessary certification of the work undertaken and receipts for moneys paid.

References and Further Reading

Chapter 1
World Health Organisation: International Classification of Functioning, Disability and Health, 2001.

Chapter 2
J. Fiske et al, *British Dental Journal,* 1998.
Elisabeth Kübler-Ross, *On Death and Dying*, 1969.
Miguel de Cervantes, Don Quixote, Walker Books, 2009.
A. del Valle and M. Romero, 'Don Quixote's Countenance Before and After Losing His Teeth', *Journal of Dental Research,* February 2009.
David Harris et al, 'A Comparison of Implant-retained Mandibular Overdentures and Conventional Dentures on Quality of Life in Edentulous Patients: a Randomized, Prospective, Within-subject Controlled Clinical Trial', *Clinical Oral Implants Research*, 2013.

Chapter 3
National Census for Ireland, 2006.
TILDA: The Irish LongituDinal Study on Ageing, http://www.tcd.ie/tilda.
Dr Alex Comfort, *Ageing: the Biology of Senescence*, 1964.
World Health Organisation: *International Classification of Functioning, Disability and Health*, 2001.
Professor Finbar Allen, 'Nutritional Status of Edentulous Patients at the Cork Dental School and Hospital', 2005.
'Café Coronary', *The Irish Times*, Thursday, 16 June 2011.

Roger E. Mittleman, MD and Charles V. Wetli, MD, 'The Fatal Café Coronary', *The Journal of the American Medical Association,*1982.

Dr R. Wick, 'Review of Victims Seen at Autopsy', *Journal of Forensic Medicine*, 2006.

Oral Health Services Research Centre, University College Cork, *National Survey of Adult Dental Health*, 2000-2002.

National Council on Ageing and Older People (NCAOP), www.welfare.ie/en/downloads/ncaop.pdf.

Chapter 5

Hugh Trevor-Roper, *The European Witch-Craze of the Sixteenth and Seventeenth Centuries,* 1969.

Hugh Trevor-Roper, *The Crisis of the Seventeenth Century,* 1967.

Stephanie Pain, 'The Great Tooth Robbery', *New Scientist*, 16 June 2001.

Nature Publishing Group and Dr Eric Cruzby, 'Roman Soldier Tooth Implant', *Nature*, Vol. 391, January 1988.

Malcolm Gladwell, *The Tipping Point: How Little Things Can Make a Big Difference, 2000.*

Chapter 6

Mouth Cancer Awareness Day, www.mouthcancerawareness.ie.

Chapter 7

Elaine Williams-McClarence, *A Matter Of Balance,* Goteborg, 1992.

Brånemark P.-I. et al, *Tissue Integrated Prostheses, Osseointegration in Clinical Dentistry,* Quintessence, 1985

Chapter 9

David Harris in *The Brånemark Novum Protocol for Same-Day Teeth: A Global Perspective*, Quintessence, 2001.

David Harris in Worthington and Brånemark, *Advanced Osseointegration Surgery*, Quintessence, 1992.

Chapter 10

Irish Dental Council, 'Choosing Your Dentist at Home or Abroad', www.dentalcouncil.ie/choosingyourdentist.php.

Irish Dental Council, 'Code of Practice Relating to Infection Control in Dentistry', www.dentalcouncil.ie/g_crossinfection.php.

Commission on Dental Accreditation in Canada (CDAC), https://www.cda-adc.ca.

Index